Marcelo Sebastião Rezende

Avian flu, migratory birds and poultry health

Marcelo Sebastião Rezende

Avian flu, migratory birds and poultry health

A case of sanitary control in commercial and subsistence poultry farming

ScienciaScripts

Imprint
Any brand names and product names mentioned in this book are subject to trademark, brand or patent protection and are trademarks or registered trademarks of their respective holders. The use of brand names, product names, common names, trade names, product descriptions etc. even without a particular marking in this work is in no way to be construed to mean that such names may be regarded as unrestricted in respect of trademark and brand protection legislation and could thus be used by anyone.

Cover image: www.ingimage.com

This book is a translation from the original published under ISBN 978-613-9-67840-2.

Publisher:
Sciencia Scripts
is a trademark of
Dodo Books Indian Ocean Ltd. and OmniScriptum S.R.L publishing group

120 High Road, East Finchley, London, N2 9ED, United Kingdom
Str. Armeneasca 28/1, office 1, Chisinau MD-2012, Republic of Moldova, Europe
Printed at: see last page
ISBN: 978-620-8-18163-5

SUMMARY

1 INTRODUCTION 2
2 METHODOLOGY 6
3 Results and discussion 14
4 SANITARY DEFENSE SYSTEM FOR THE PREVENTION AND CONTROL OF AVIAN INFLUENZA 57
5 FINAL CONSIDERATIONS 66
6 REFERENCES 68
ANNEX A 75

1 INTRODUCTION

Brazilian poultry has a leading position in chicken meat production worldwide, producing 11.032 million tons in 2008. This figure represents 15.5% of the world's production, estimated at 71.249 million tons. The volume is quite representative in that, over seven years, it gives an increase of 63.77% in the annual production of chicken meat in Brazil, while the world average increased by 36.29%. In terms of exports, the figures are even more representative, since the country exported 3.242 million tons of chicken meat in 2008, representing 38.61% of world exports. This figure consolidates the country as the world's largest exporter, a position it has held since 2004 (ABEF, 2009).

Chicken meat is one of the main products on the Brazilian agribusiness export agenda. This prominent position is due to a number of factors, including the advances made in genetics, nutrition, handling, ambience and, above all, health control, which have undoubtedly enabled Brazil to make great strides in the global market (ABEF, 2009).

However, in recent years, we have seen the occurrence of various diseases in animals that also affect humans. Called zoonoses, these diseases, such as Mad Cow Disease and Avian Influenza, have aroused enormous concern among the world's scientific community, national governments and the general public. Recent studies have shown that the so-called emerging diseases have quadrupled in the last 50 years, 60% of which are associated with transmission between humans and animals (JONES et al., 2008). The United States Agency for International Development (USAID) has launched a five-year global program to train people to identify and combat outbreaks of new emerging diseases, such as Influenza A (H1N1). The project, called -Respond", which has an initial budget of U$185 million, will employ an integrated approach that brings together public and private sector organizations to combat emerging diseases on a global scale (WORLD POULTRY, 2009).

Throughout history, there have been several flu pandemics. There was the Spanish flu at the beginning of the 20th century, the Asian flu (1957 to 1963) and the Hong Kong flu (1968 to 1970). The Spanish Flu is considered the worst pandemic of all time, wiping out between 40 and 100 million people worldwide; the Asian Flu killed around two million people and the Hong Kong Flu around one million people. These pandemics were characterized by high mortality among young people; evolution in epidemic waves, the first being milder and the others more severe; higher transmission rates than seasonal flu and regional heterogeneity, justified by the complexity of the immunological characteristics of the inhabitants, the subtypes of the circulating viruses and the geographical and climatic details of the affected areas (MILLER et al., 2009).

The subtype of the virus that caused the Spanish flu is the same as the one that caused the recent swine flu, initially called H1N1. Há studies indicate that the Influenza A virus is descended from the virus that caused the Spanish Flu, but, for the time being, with a lower mortality potential (FAUCI et al., 2009).

Accentuating since 2003, Avian Influenza has affected several countries in Europe, Africa and especially Asia, causing the death of hundreds of people and the sacrifice of thousands of birds around the world (WHO, 2009a).

There are some characteristics that differentiate swine flu from avian flu. The main subtypes of the virus that cause avian flu are H5N1 and H7N7, while in swine flu it is the H1N1 subtype. The spread of Avian Influenza occurs through direct contact with birds, or their excrement and secretions, while in Influenza A it occurs from person to person (WHO, 2009). The spread of Influenza A is much faster and more widespread, affecting 208 countries by December 2009, causing the death of more than 9,500 people worldwide (WHO, 2009f).

Avian Influenza has caused great concern in the world's scientific community as it has a lethality rate of approximately 60% in the human population, although it has a lower transmission capacity than the others. Although it is exotic in Brazil, the risk of its appearance must be considered, given the existence of migratory routes for birds coming from affected regions, mainly North America. Some epidemiological studies in Brazil have revealed the occurrence of migratory birds carrying the low pathogenic avian influenza virus (LPAI) (AZEVEDO JÙNIOR, 2006).

The avifauna survey carried out around the Amador Aguiar I and II Hydroelectric Power Plants in the municipalities of Uberlândia, Araguari and Indianópolis made it possible to identify four species of migratory birds from North America (MANNA and TOLEDO, 2008). The rural survey carried out by the Municipal Department of Agriculture and Supply of the Uberlândia City Hall showed that in the rural area of the municipality of Uberlândia, the majority of rural producers keep chickens and hens at home as a subsistence system, lacking the technology to guarantee the health of their flocks.

The municipality of Uberlândia-MG is an important center for poultry production and genetics, with industrial breeding systems for heavy, semi-heavy and light breeders, broiler chickens, laying hens and turkeys, as well as a modern production system for *specific pathogen* free (*SPF)* eggs, which are used for the production of human and veterinary vaccines, as well as being used in laboratories for diagnosing various diseases (REZENDE et al., 2008). One of the characteristics of these farms is the use of biosecurity measures to prevent the introduction of diseases into their plantations, whose population represents more than 99% of the total number of broiler chickens and hens in the municipality. The Rural Survey of rural Uberlândia indicated that some subsistence farms are close to industrial farms. The complex formed by the occurrence of migratory birds from regions where avian influenza has occurred, present in the same environment as subsistence birds, which lack biosecurity measures, and their proximity to industrial farms, creates a risk of transmission that must be considered, with economic and public health impacts.

Brazil has its own legislation, Normative Instruction 17 of April 7, 2006, which regulates the contingency plan in the event of Avian Influenza. The plan is structured at federal and state level, with responsibilities shared between the public and private sectors. In addition, training has been given to technicians in the public and private sector, in order to prepare them for the possible occurrence of Avian Influenza. Human and material resources must be taken into account if the disease is to be successfully controlled. The characterization of the animal health and public health systems at federal, state and municipal level shows the need for better structuring in terms of greater active and passive surveillance capacity and an efficient response in a contingency situation.

The recent outbreaks of H1N1 flu (August to October 2009) in the municipality of Uberlândia have put the municipality's hospitals on alert for more complex situations. There were difficulties in finding ICU places for patients with proven or suspected infections. The city currently has just over 630,000 inhabitants, with 1,226 hospital beds, giving an average of 1.94 beds per 1,000 inhabitants. This figure is lower than the average for Brazil, which is 2.4 (UBERLÂNDIA, 2009).

1.1 Objectives

1.1.1 General Objective

The general objective of this work is to present the possibility of Avian Influenza transmission in the municipality of Uberlândia, considering an epidemiological model that involves the presence of migratory birds and the domestic population of chickens, hens and turkeys.

1.1.20 bjectives

The specific objectives were:

a) To list and characterize the northern migratory species that occur around the Amador Aguiar I and II hydroelectric dams, identified in the birdlife survey carried out by the company Manno e Toledo Planejamento Ambiental Ltda, at the request of the Capim Branco Energy Consortium;

b) Mapping rural properties with poultry in the rural area of the municipality of Uberlândia, especially those close to the Amador Aguiar I and II reservoirs, identifying their distances and the number of birds present, through the rural survey of the Municipal Department of Agriculture and Supply of the Uberlândia City Hall;

c) To identify the main shortcomings in the biosecurity of chicken and hen farms, or subsistence farms, which can facilitate the entry and spread of specific diseases that can be transmitted to humans;

d) Present the public health defense system and the means of control of private initiative with regard to the prevention of the occurrence of avian influenza and the contingency plan, admitting its introduction into the country.

2 METHODOLOGY

2.1 General Characteristics of the Study Area

The municipality of Uberlândia is located in the Triângulo Mineiro mesoregion, in the southwestern part of the state of Minas Gerais, in the southeastern region of Brazil (UBERLÂNDIA, 2009). The municipality is bounded by the geographical coordinates of 18°30' - 19°30' south latitude and 47°50' - 48°50' west longitude of Greenwich, at an average altitude of 900m, with an area of around 4,115 km^2 (ASSUNÇÂO; LIMA; ROSA, 1991).

The climate of the Triângulo Mineiro region, according to the Koppen climate classification, is of the Aw type, characterized by a dry winter and a rainy summer, dominated predominantly by intertropical and polar systems. Temperatures vary on average from 19°C to 27°C, with an average rainfall of around 1500 mm/year. The rainy season generally begins in October and ends in April, with the highest rainfall in December and January. The dry season lasts from May to September (SILVA; ASSUNÇÂO, 2004).

Located in the Plateaus and Chapadas of the Paranà Sedimentary Basin, the municipality of Uberlândia is part of the Southern Plateau sub-unit of the Paranà Basin (Radam/Brazil/83), characterized by being tabular, slightly undulating, with an altitude of less than 1,000 m (UBERLANDIA, 2008).

The soils are acidic, of the latosol type, predominantly red-yellow and sandy-clayey. In the western part of the municipality, at altitudes ranging from 700 to 850 m, the soils are shallower, with patches of red-yellow podzolic type and low fertility. The predominant vegetation here is sub-caducifolia forest. In the vicinity of the urban area, the relief is more undulating, with altitudes ranging from 800 to 900 m. The rivers and streams flow over the basalt, with several waterfalls and rapids, where the soils are fertile, of the red and dark red latosol type. The slopes are gentle, generally less than 30%. In the northern part, close to the Araguari River Valley, the landscape has a strongly undulating relief, with an altitude of 800 to 1,000 m and patches of very fertile soil, of the dark red latosol and podzolic type. The characteristic vegetation is cerrado, and its main physiognomic types are vereda, campo limpo, campo sujo or cerradinho, cerradao, mata de vàrzea, mata de galeria or ciliar and mata mesofitica (SANO; ALMEIDA, 1998).

The municipality has 219.00 km^2 of urban area and 3,896.822 km^2 of rural area, totaling 4,115.822 km2 (UBERLÂNDIA, 2009).

The municipality of Uberlândia is drained by the Tijuco River and Araguari River basins, both tributaries of the Paranaiba River (UBERLÂNDIA, 2009).

The Araguari river basin covers the eastern part of the municipality. Its main tributary in the area of the municipality is the Uberabinha River, which passes through the city of Uberlândia. The potential of the Araguari River is already being exploited, with the Nova Ponte hydroelectric power station 80 km away, the Miranda power station 20 km away and the Capim Branco power station 10 km away (UBERLÂNDIA, 2009).

The estimated population of Uberlândia, based on the demographic census of the Brazilian Institute of Geography and Statistics (IBGE) for 2007, is 608,369 inhabitants, with the urban population accounting for 97.5% of the total (UBERLÂNDIA, 2009).

The municipality's economic activity is carried out by 28,686 establishments, of which 1,374 are in the primary sector, 3,425 in the secondary sector and 23,887 in the tertiary sector. These sectors accounted for 1.8%, 50.2% and 48.2% respectively of ICMS revenue in 2006 (UBERLÂNDIA, 2009).

2.2 Organization and Analysis of Research Data

This work was prepared using information obtained from the rural survey of the municipality of Uberlândia, carried out by the Municipal Department of Agriculture and Supply, and from the list of birds recorded at the Amador Aguiar I and II hydroelectric power stations, It is an integral part of the final report of the "Project to Confirm the Presence of Threatened Species at the Amador Aguiar I and II HPPs", carried out by the company Manna e Toledo Planejamento Ambiental Ltda, hired by the Capim Branco Energia Consortium (CCBE). This project is part of the program to monitor endangered Alate and Terrestrial fauna in the area surrounding the reservoirs of the power plants (MANNA E TOLEDO, 2008).

CCBE holds the concession to operate the Amador Aguiar I and II HPPs.

The Rural Survey of the Municipality of Uberlândia was carried out between June and October 2006, by collecting data and detailed information on the socio-economic and productive conditions of the agricultural sector on rural properties in the municipality of Uberlândia. The aim was to obtain a database that would provide a precise diagnosis for drawing up proposals and programs aimed at the real needs of the local agricultural complex.

The work carried out by the Municipal Department of Agriculture and Supply consisted of *on-site* visits to 2,784 rural properties in the municipality, georeferencing them. Covering an area of 367,978.51 ha, representing 94.4% of the total rural area, 3,260 rural producers were interviewed. The survey was based on filling in a detailed questionnaire about the property, the farming activities carried out and the people living there.

The area surveyed did not include district headquarters, leisure cottages, fishing ranches, roadside gas stations and roads.

In order to carry out the work, the Uberlândia City Council spent R$146,204.24 on the purchase of microcomputers, GPS, snacks, booklets, hiring staff and renting vehicles.

The rural survey involved 12 census takers, four monitors (agricultural technicians), four drivers, five typists, a field coordinator, an administrative coordinator and a general coordinator, all of whom were employed by the municipality of Uberlândia (Figure 1).

The results of the research were compiled in tables and graphs presented in the textual part of the paper. Using the data provided, it was possible to identify the land ownership structure, the conditions of possession and occupation of the rural space, the agricultural activities carried out and the population's schooling and age data.

By locating the properties, obtained through georeferencing, surveying the number of birds present on the properties, the type of farming carried out (commercial, industrial or subsistence) and the species involved (chicken, hens and turkeys), it was possible to draw up a map of the distribution of poultry farms in the municipality of Uberlândia (Map 1). The basic data for the map came from the Municipal Planning and Environment Department (SEPLAMA), the Municipal Water and Sewage Department (DMAE), the Supply and Agriculture Department (SEDUR) and Geoprocessing in Minas Gerais (GEOMINAS), using CBERS satellite images to vectorize the boundaries of the reservoirs in the municipality of Uberlândia. The software used was ESRI's ARCGIS, at a scale of 1:125,000.

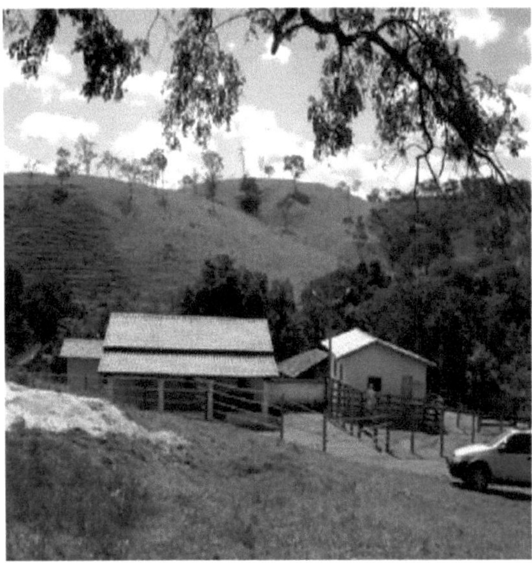

Figure 1. Rural survey. Visits to rural properties in the municipality of Uberlândia - MG, 2006.

Source: SEGATO (2006).

The avifauna survey was carried out in the riparian environments of the Araguari River, whose basin covers an area of approximately 21,856 km^2 , formed by 20 municipalities in the state of Minas Gerais. Extending for 475 km, the Araguari River rises in the Serra da Canastra National Park, in the municipality of Sao Roque de Minas, and is one of the main tributaries of the Paranaiba River. At the confluence of the states of Minas Gerais, Sao Paulo and Mato Grosso do Sul, the Paranaiba River meets the Grande River, forming the transnational Paranà River basin (BACCARO et al., 2003).

The Araguari River has a high energy potential, represented by the Nova Ponte (80 km from the city of Uberlândia), Miranda (20 km from the city of Uberlândia) and Amador Aguiar I and II hydroelectric plants, located 20 and 48 km from the city of Uberlândia, respectively (UBERLÂNDIA, 2009).

Riparian environments were chosen at random from the native riverside vegetation of the Amador Aguiar I and II hydroelectric power stations (Figure 2). The first incursion was aimed at recognizing and selecting the areas and in the 13 subsequent campaigns, systematic studies were carried out to sample the avifauna.

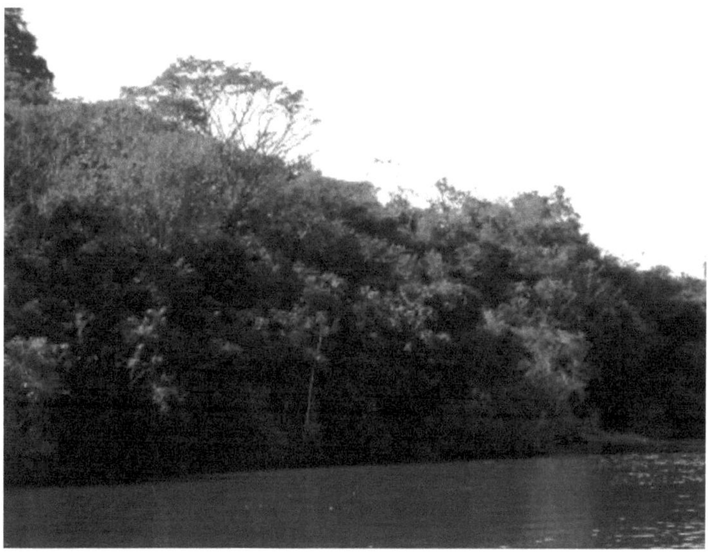

Figure 2 - Vegetation on the banks of the Amador Aguiar I hydroelectric dam.

Source: REZENDE (2009).

Three 2.0 km long transects were established in four locations in the study area, parallel to the riparian vegetation of the Araguari River. The transects were marked with ribbons every 200 meters, totaling at least 10 equidistant points. Trails of 200 meters were also opened in each area to place mist nets.

Three complementary methods were used to collect data on wild bird fauna: sampling by listening points, sampling by direct observation and sampling with mist nets.

Observations were made with binoculars (10X42 mm) and recordings with a portable recorder (Marantz PMD222) with the aid of a directional microphone (Senheiser ME67). Field guides were used to identify the species visually and acoustically by comparison with the recordings. The scientific nomenclature was used in accordance with the resolutions established by the Brazilian Committee of Ornithological Records.

The bird species were separated by type of habit, food guild, status (endemic, threatened), commercial value (game) and/or domestic value (xerimbabo), potential pollinators or seed dispersers (indicators of environmental quality) and sensitivity.

For species threatened with extinction in the state of Minas Gerais, we followed the Normative Decision of the State Council for Environmental Policy of Minas Gerais (COPAM) No. 041/95, of December 20, 1995, at the national level, the Normative Instruction of the Ministry of the Environment No. 3, of May 27, 2003 and at the global level the list proposed by the World Conservation Union (IUCN).

The feeding guilds considered were for nectarivorous, carnivorous, omnivorous, granivorous, frugivorous and insectivorous species.

For the habitat classification, the species were divided into aquatic, essentially and exclusively grassland and essentially and exclusively forest.

The species were classified in terms of their sensitivity to anthropogenic disturbances as high, medium and low sensitivity. Sensitivity to disturbances can evaluate the species as an indicator of environmental quality. Thus, areas with a greater number of species with high sensitivity may indicate that the site is in a good state of conservation.

Sampling points were established in each area and their application consisted of setting up a network of points in the habitat. The observer remained at each point for seven minutes in the morning, recording all the species observed and heard, with the points spaced 200 meters apart.

In direct observation sampling, non-inear transects were walked in each area, carried out at a slow pace by the observer, in order to visually and/or aurally record all the species found. This method was used during all periods of the day, where *playback* techniques were also employed, focusing mainly on the noises of endangered, rare and endemic bird species.

When sampling with *mist* nets, 13 to 15 mist nets 12m long and 2.8m high were used, preferably set in a linear sequence, making up 200-250 meters in length. The nets were set up from dawn until dusk.

All the birds captured were tagged with metal rings supplied by the National Research Centre for the Conservation of Wild Birds (CEMAVE), a decentralized unit of the Chico Mendes Institute for Biodiversity Conservation (ICMBIO). The capture, tagging and recapture method allows each bird to receive an individual code, capable of identifying it when it is recaptured.

2.3 Simulated Exercise on the Introduction of the Highly Pathogenic Avian Influenza Virus in the State of Minas Gerais

With the aim of training professionals from the official federal and state defense agencies, as well as those from the private sector, representing the main poultry production companies in Minas Gerais, a course and simulated exercise was held to eradicate exotic and emergency poultry diseases. The course, organized by the Ministry of Agriculture, Livestock and Supply in partnership with the Instituto Mineiro de Agropecuària, took place from 15 to 20 October 2007, in the municipality of Uberaba-MG.

The event was coordinated and guided by five people, bringing together a group of 33 participants from different regions of the state, as well as representatives from Brasilia, the Federal District.

The first stage of the program included lectures on the biological, epidemiological, economic, social and environmental aspects of avian influenza, as well as control models adopted in countries affected by the disease.

Two simulations were carried out, in the office and in the field, to practice the concepts learned in the lectures.

The cabinet simulation took place on the premises of the event. The participants were divided into four groups and a coordinator was chosen for each team. To carry out the activity, a hypothetical case of AI was presented, adopting an epidemiological model to identify the outbreaks where the disease would occur. This exercise considered the interdiction of outbreaks, the adoption of sanitary barriers, the installation of systems for disinfecting materials and vehicles, the sacrifice of poultry and pigs from properties, the elimination of waste generated, the sanitation of properties and the sanitary vacuum. Consideration was given to the adoption of protective measures through the delimitation of protection zones (3 km) and surveillance zones (10 km) and the planning of transportation logistics such as access for residents and the movement of vehicles. The costs inherent in the procedure were also taken into account, including personnel costs, the purchase of products such as fuel, vehicles and sanitizing materials, and compensation for the animals sacrificed. Another aspect considered was the need to issue a clarification note as a result of the press reports. It is worth highlighting the intensive use of satellite images (Figure 3) and geographic coordinates during all phases of the control program. At the end of the work, a presentation was made to all the participants.

For the field simulation, the training participants were divided into three groups. Each team was given an investigation and an epidemiological model of an outbreak of avian influenza, hypothetically occurring in the municipality of Uberaba, Minas Gerais. In this case, with a list of the properties involved and their respective geographical coordinates, the groups carried out field visits.

During the field visits, the teams had the opportunity to gather information and the specific conditions of the properties in which to carry out the work. With the information gathered, the teams carried out the actions at the course site, using the strategies they had practiced in the previous exercise. At the end of the activity, the groups gave their presentations.

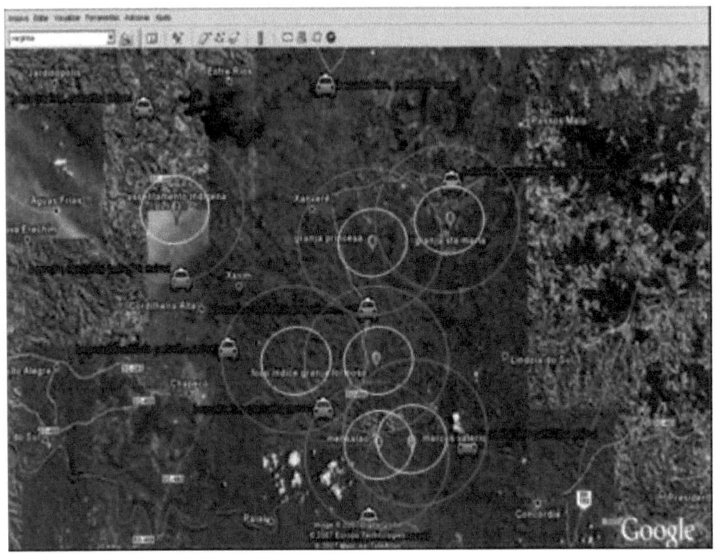

Figure 3 - Satellite image used in the Emergency Exotic Disease Simulation Course in Uberaba-MG, 2007.

Source: Exotic Disease Simulation Course in Uberaba-MG (2007).

As a complement to the activities of the simulation course, there was training in the collection of material for laboratory diagnosis and a study to assess the risks of introducing the highly pathogenic virus into the state of Minas Gerais, according to the regions of the state.

At the end of the training, the potential risks of the introduction of avian influenza in the Triângulo Mineiro region were listed, which are considered in the discussion of this paper.

In order to discuss and substantiate the results of the research data, it was essential to use the theoretical framework, using books related to the research topic, scientific articles, atlases and consultations of specific sites on the World Wide Web.

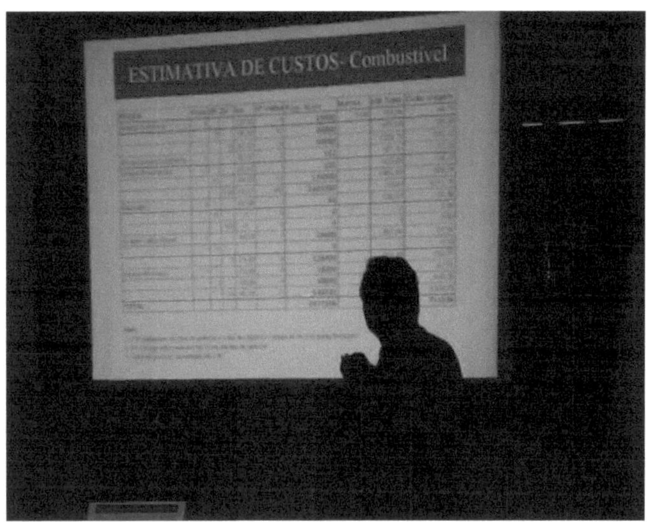

Figure 4 - Presentation of the Exotic and Emergency Disease Simulation Course exercise in Uberaba, 2007.

Source: Exotic Disease Simulation Course in Uberaba-MG (2007).

3 RESULTS AND DISCUSSION

3.1 Rural Survey of the Municipality of Uberlândia

The municipality of Uberlândia has a total area of 411,582.2 ha, of which 21,900 ha are urban and 389,682.2 are rural (Graph 1) (UBERLÂNDIA, 2008). The aim of the survey was to set up a database to provide a precise diagnosis for drawing up proposals and programs geared to the real needs of the local agricultural complex.

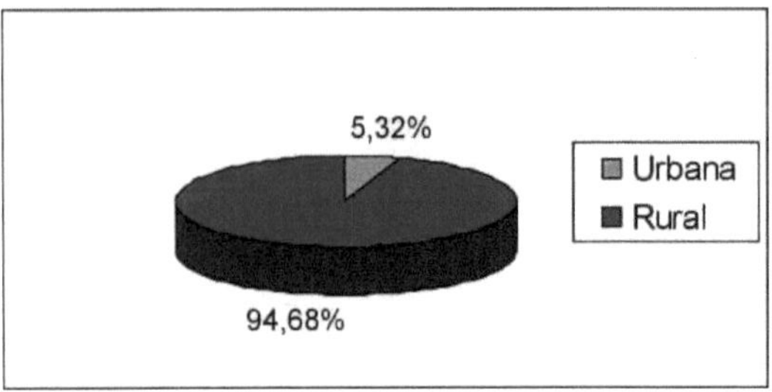

Graph 1 - Urban and rural areas of the municipality of Uberlândia.

Source: Rural survey, 2006.

Adapted from REZENDE (2009).

The visits covered 94.43% of the total rural area. The area surveyed did not include district headquarters, leisure cottages, fishing ranches and roadside gas stations (Graph 2).

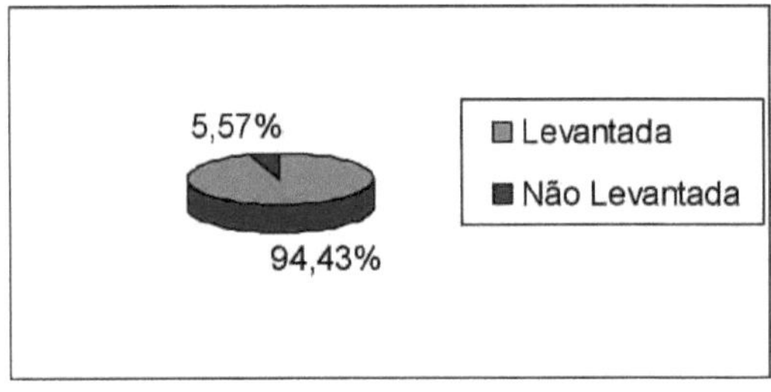

Graph 2 - Rural area of the municipality of Uberlândia covered by the rural survey.

Source: Rural survey, 2006.

Adapted from REZENDE (2009).

The survey showed an extremely concentrated land ownership structure of the surveyed rural area, where 68.7% of properties up to 80 ha occupy 14% of the total area, while 9.9% of properties over 300 ha account for 60.7% of the total area (Table 1).

Table 1

Land stratification of the rural area surveyed in the municipality of Uberlândia - MG, 2006.

Stratification	Properties	%	Area (ha)	(%)
0-20 ha	870	31,3	11.186	3,0
20-80 ha	1043	37,5	40.333	11,0
80-300 ha	594	21,3	93.137	25,3
> 300 ha	277	9,9	223.322	60,7
TOTAL	2.784	100,0	367.978	100,0

Source: Rural survey, 2006 Adapted: REZENDE (2009).

The rural survey also showed the ownership conditions of the properties, according to their size, as illustrated in Table 2. The majority of rural producers are owners themselves (66.01%), with a greater share of larger properties - over 300 ha (87.66%) and a smaller share of smaller properties (up to 20 ha), with 52.90%. Settled producers account for 19.39% of the total, with 32.65% and 25.21% respectively in smallholdings (up to 20 ha) and small properties (20.1 - 80 ha). Leaseholders account for 14.60% of all producers, with a larger share in medium-sized properties (80.1 - 300 ha), at 19.40%.

Table 2

Tenure conditions of rural producers in the municipality of Uberlândia - MG, 2006.

	Types of Producers							
Property size (ha)	Tenants	%	Settlers	%	Owners	%	Total	%
0-20	147	14,45	332	32,65	538	52,90	1017	100
20,1 - 80	147	12,35	300	25,21	743	62,44	1190	100
80,1 - 300	143	19,40	-	-	594	80,60	737	100
Above 300	39	12,34	-	-	277	87,66	316	100
Total	476	14,60	632	19,39	2152	66,01	3260	100

Source: Rural survey, 2006.

Adapted from REZENDE (2009).

The rural properties in the municipality are characterized in Table 3. Livestock farming occupies 34.66% of the municipality's area and is carried out on 1,750 properties.

Table 3

Characterization of rural properties in the municipality of Uberlândia - MG

Activity	*No. of properties*	*Area (ha)*	*% in relation to the area of the municipality*
Livestock	1750	127569,09	34,66
Agriculture	1363	70533,98	19,17
Legal reserve	2397	64643,50	17,57
Unused Area	865	27952,48	7,60
Leased Area	424	47433,88	12,90
APP	2088	18430,42	5,00
Improvements	2442	4708,17	1,28
Cerrado/Campo	148	4581,07	1,24
Unused Area	170	1458,70	0,40
Invaded Area	2	616,27	0,17
Donated Area	1	30,95	0,01

Source: Rural survey, 2006.

Adapted from REZENDE (2009).

Livestock activities include poultry farming, cattle farming, goat farming, sheep farming and pig farming (Table 4). The livestock numbers for the municipality of Uberlândia are shown in Table 4. The rural survey found that 1,423 of the total number of farmers interviewed (43.7%) keep poultry on their properties.

Table 4

Livestock activities carried out by the producers interviewed

Activity	No. of producers	%	Hosted staff
Poultry farming	1.423	43,7	6.612.108
Bovine farming	2.157	66,2	200.886
Goat farming	36	1,1	399
Equine farming	1.218	37,4	4.454
Sheep farming	51	1,6	4.831
Pig farming	913	28,0	213.691

The profile of the producers reveals an age group above 30 (Table 5), where 60.21% of those interviewed are between 31 and 60 years old. The average age is 48.

Table 5

Age group of producers interviewed

Age	No. of producers	%
Up to 30 years old	168	5,15
31 to 60 years	1963	60,21
Over 60	898	27,55
No information	231	7,09
Total	3260	100,00

Source: Rural survey, 2006.

Adapted from REZENDE (2009).

Table 6 shows the education level of producers, where the majority (1210 producers - 37.10%) have incomplete primary education.

Table 6

Level of education of the producers interviewed

Education	No. of producers	%
1st grade incomplete	1210	37,12
1st grade completed	502	15,40
2nd degree	539	16,53
Technical level	74	2,27
3rd grade	695	21,32
No schooling	78	2,39
No reply	162	4,97

Total	3260	100,00

Source: Rural survey, 2006.

Adapted from REZENDE (2009).

Assessing the profile of rural residents, there were a total of 9,433 people, predominantly aged over 18 (Table 7). The percentage of owners and family members represents 41.07% of rural residents, while the percentage of employees and family members is 58.93%.

Table 7

Age group of rural residents in the municipality of Uberlândia

Age group	Owners and their families	Employees and their families	Total	% of residents
Up to 6 years	188	348	536	5,68
6 - 12 years	293	402	695	7,37
12 - 18 years	334	324	658	6,98
Over 18	3059	4485	7544	79,97
Total	3874	5559	9433	100,00

Source: Rural survey, 2006.

Adapted from REZENDE (2009).

There were 7,875 workers employed in the fields, of which 4,725 (60.00%) were permanent workers, 2,284 (29.00%) were family workers and 473 (6.00%) were temporary workers.

Considering the level of professional training of producers, only 37% have already taken part in a training course, while 45% revealed that they have no interest in taking part in this type of event.

Evaluating the type of water source used on rural properties, the main source was local surface water, including streams, mines, gullies, dams and rivers (Table 8).

Table 8

Water sources in rural properties in the municipality of Uberlândia, 2006.

Type of font	Quantity	%
Stream	1526	54,81
Mina	1466	52,66
Watering hole	947	34,01
Cistern	734	26,36
Dam	730	26,22
Rio/Ribeirao	552	19,83
Artesian well	490	17,60
DMAE	55	1,98

Source: Rural survey, 2006.

Adapted from REZENDE (2009).

The 2006 data from the Rural Survey of the municipality of Uberlândia revealed that the poultry population in the municipality was around 6,600,000, made up of 92.2% chicken and 7.8% turkeys.

The same study indicated that the activity is carried out by 1,423 chicken producers (43.65%) and 25 turkey farmers (0.77%). Table 9 shows the classification of chicken producers according to the size of the property and the number of birds present in each situation. It can be seen that the vast majority of producers are subsistence farmers (73.01%), but they raise a small number of birds, i.e. only 0.62% of the total, concentrated mainly on smallholdings and small properties (71.89%). Although commercial and industrial producers account for 26.99% of all farmers, they make up 99.38% of the poultry flock, with typically industrial breeding taking up 98.96% of the total flock of chickens/chicken, of industrial lineage, with only 8.01% of producers.

The profile of the producers and their turkey flocks are shown in Table 10. It can be seen that there is no record of turkeys being raised for subsistence or commercial purposes, only for industrial purposes. There is also a predominance of producers with properties of up to 80 ha (80.00%), covering 53.33% of turkey farming in the municipality.

3.2 Characterization of Poultry Raising for Subsistence in the Rural Area of the Municipality of Uberlândia

Subsistence farms generally breed what are known as "caipira" poultry. These are actually chickens obtained by crossing various breeds. Until the 1960s, poultry farming in Brazil was characterized by raising chickens without any specialization or use of technology, either in the field (extensive system) or in grassy paddocks (semi-extensive). Even today, caipira chickens and eggs are part of the cuisine of various regional cultures and raising caipira poultry is still considered an excellent business for small and medium-sized owners, with excellent profitability (KISHIBE et al., 2009).

Table 9

Classification of chicken breeders and number of birds housed in Uberlândia.

Size of Property (ha)	Types of Producers					Broiler/chicken flock housed				
	Subsistence[1]	%	Commercial +[2] Industrial[3]	%	TOTAL	No. of birds - subsistence	%	No. of birds - commercial + industrial	%	TOTAL
Up to 20	343	33,01	108	28,13	451	11.669	30,83	815.686	13,46	827.355
20,1-80	404	38,88	158	41,14	562	13.547	35,79	1.814.187	29,94	1.827.734
80,1-300	209	20,12	77	20,05	286	8.771	23,17	1.700.060	28,05	1.708.831
Above 300	83	7,99	41	10,68	124	3.864	10,21	1.730.113	28,55	1.733.977
Total	1039	100,00	384	100,00	1423	37.851	100,00	6.060.046	100,00	6.097.897

Source: Rural survey, 2006.

Adapted from REZENDE (2009).

1 Own creation and consumption
2 Own breeding for commercialization
3 Creation in a partnership system

Table 10

Classification of turkey breeders and number of birds housed in Uberlândia.

Size of Property (ha)	Types of Producers					Broiler/chicken flock housed				
	Subsistence + commercial	%	Industrial	%	TOTAL	No. of birds - subsistence + commercial	%	No. of birds - industrial	%	TOTAL
Up to 20	-	-	6	24,00	6	-	-	115.741	22,51	115.741
20,1-80	-	-	14	56,00	14	-	-	158.470	30,82	158.470
80,1-300	-	-	3	12,00	3	-	-	92.000	17,89	92.000
Above 300	-	-	2	8,00	2	-	-	148.000	28,78	148.000
Total	-	-	25	100,00	25	-	-	514.211	100,00	514.211

Source: Rural survey, 2006.

Adapted from REZENDE (2009).

In subsistence farming, it is important to adopt good management and biosecurity measures, such as: a good ratio between the number of birds and the area occupied (density); the use of appropriate feeders, drinkers and nests; waste management; the use of contaminant-free water; a balanced diet; vaccinations and the adoption of measures to protect against diseases (KISHIBE et al., 2009).

The rural survey showed that the vast majority of subsistence poultry farms do not comply with minimum biosecurity standards. The birds are raised in the field, exposed to contact with birds and other wild birds, and do not receive a nutritionally balanced diet. The main source of water used, including for watering the birds, comes from surface water (Table 8), without any form of microbiocidal treatment.

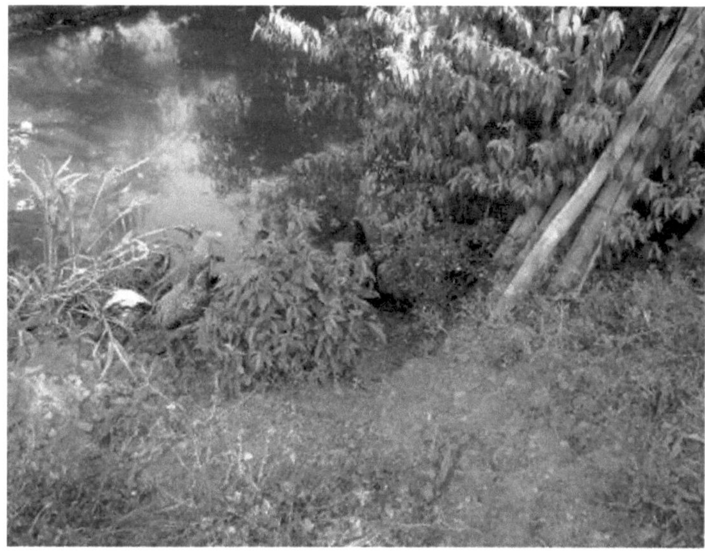

Figure 5 - Caipira birds raised on the banks of the Amador Aguiar I hydroelectric dam.

Source: REZENDE, 2009.

Another relevant piece of information is the lack of concern or ignorance on the part of producers regarding the possibility of diseases occurring in poultry flocks, since, according to the Rural Survey, 99.5% of producers do not use any type of vaccine as a preventative procedure.

The rural survey also showed that a significant proportion of producers, around 55%, have no interest in improving their professional skills.

Map 1 shows the distribution of poultry farms (chickens and turkeys) in the municipality of Uberlândia, based on the Rural Survey. It shows the predominance of free-range farming. Another important factor is the proximity of subsistence and commercial farms to industrial farms. The proximity of these farms to industrial farms, which are significantly larger in terms of the number of birds, represents a risk for the transmission and perpetuation of avian diseases in the region. Table 11 shows the distances between industrial farms and subsistence and/or commercial farms, with the population of birds involved (REZENDE; SILVA; LIMA, 2008).

Some diseases identified in free-range poultry found in rural areas of the city are typical of farms that do not adopt minimum biosecurity measures, such as infections associated with *Mycoplasma gallisepticum, Mycoplasma synoviae, Salmonella pullorum and Salmonella gallinarum* (PEREIRA; SILVA, 2005ab). If wild birds were to become infected with the Avian Influenza virus, with the possibility of transmission to poultry and industrial farms, there would be a risk of the disease spreading between the birds and the human population involved in these farms.

Table 11

Distance between industrial and subsistence (caipira) farms in the municipality of Uberlândia.

Distance (m)	Creation Industrial	No. of birds	Creation Caipira	No. of birds
0 - 100	4	147.500	4	215
101 - 500	17	423.800	23	935
501-1000	50	1.861.575	107	5.618
1001-1500	72	3.821.236	157	7.747
1501-2000	76	4.571.736	185	9.218
2001-2500	76	4.813.889	268	12.339
2501-3000	82	4.685.420	310	17.398

Source: Rural survey, 2006.

Adapted from REZENDE (2009).

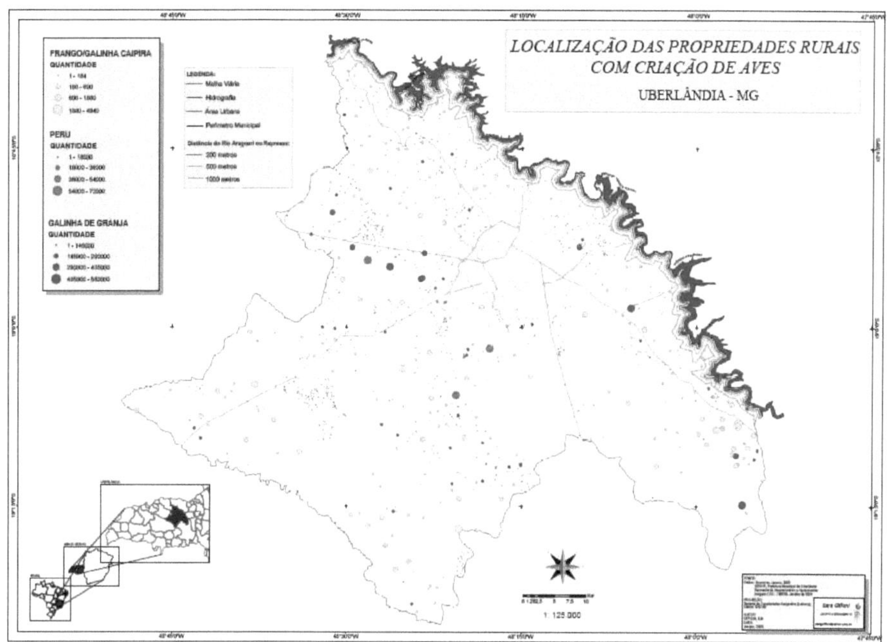

Map 1 - Distribution of poultry farms in the municipality of Uberlândia.

3.3 Characterization of Industrial Poultry Farming in the Rural Area of the Municipality of Uberlândia

The industrial breeding system includes the breeding of reproductive birds by large companies located in the municipality of Uberlândia and the breeding of chickens in a partnership system. This system, led by the agro-industries, is the system that owns the entire production process, from the production of the fertile egg to slaughter, including the marketing of the products. It was developed in the United States of America (USA) and introduced in Brazil in the 1970s (MENDES; SALDANHA, 2004). The partnership or integration system is a contractual agreement where the integrator is a company or cooperative that provides the birds at a young age (for day-old chickens), the breed (which represents approximately 70% of the production cost), technical and veterinary assistance, including vaccines and medicines. The partner or integrated company provides the facility, the equipment needed to raise the birds and the labor. In this agreement, the integrator undertakes to absorb all the birds at the end of the rearing period, with the payment of a rent to the integrated company (COTTA, 2003).

The rural survey of the municipality of Uberlândia showed that 99.38% of its poultry is kept in the industrial breeding system. Due to the demands of consumer markets and official animal protection agencies, this system meets most, if not all, of the biosecurity measures.

According to data provided by a poultry integrating company in the municipality of Uberlândia, there are 47 active integrated properties for the production of broilers, with a housing capacity of 2,400,000 birds, and 52 properties for the production of turkeys, with a housing capacity of 420,000 birds. Almost all of the poultry houses on these properties have a protected water source, water treatment, screens that prevent wild birds from gaining access and no other domestic birds (Table 12).

It should be noted that industrial poultry farms must comply with the country's and state's health legislation. It is a set of rules that establish strict requirements for location, type of construction, maintenance of health status, movement and destination of poultry, as well as criteria for the destination of by-products of the activity (BRASIL, 2007).

Table 12

Biosecurity parameters for farms in partnership with an Integrating Company in Uberlândia, 2009.

Animal Species	Protected water source	%	Chlorinate d water	%	Anti-bird screen	%	Presence of other domestic birds	%
Chicken	45/47	95,74	46/47	96,87	45/47	95,74	0/47	0,00
Turkeys	51/52	98,08	52/52	100,00	52/52	100,00	0/52	0,00

Source: Empresa Integradora, 2009.

Adapted from REZENDE (2009).

3.4 Survey of the Avifauna Surrounding the Amador Aguiar I and II Hydroelectric Power Plants

According to data from the Brazilian Committee of Ornithological Records (CBRO), *there are* 1822 species of birds recorded in Brazil, with the last update on October 5, 2008. The number of resident species comprises 1614 specimens (88.58%), of which 229 (12.56%) are considered endemic species[4] . For migratory species[5] there are 64 visitors from the northern hemisphere (3.51%), 41 from the southern hemisphere (2.25%) and six from the eastern part of Brazil (0.33%) (CBRO, 2008).

The study carried out in aquatic environments in Uberlândia, Minas Gerais, by surveying the avifauna of four lagoons in the municipality, suggests that the richness of the avifauna is related to the quality, but not the size, of the lagoons. The quality of the pond is more directly linked to the preservation of its surroundings, suggesting that its preservation has a direct influence on the number of avian species

4 Resident or sedentary species are those that reproduce in the place in question and do not originate from other places. Endemic species, included in the group of resident species, have a more restricted distribution, representing species that occur exclusively in Brazil (SICK, 1988).

5 Migratory or visiting species are those that reproduce in a given country and periodically or accidentally reach other countries (SICK, 1988).

present (BORGES; RODRIGUES; MELO, 2008).

A survey of the avifauna found at the Amador Aguiar I and II hydroelectric power plants (HPPs) between the municipalities of Uberlândia, Araguari and Indianópolis, recorded 312 species of wild birds. The species found represent 17.12% of the total number of birds occurring in Brazil. A total of 308 (98.72%) resident birds were recorded, of which seven were considered endemic (2.17%) and four migratory species from the northern hemisphere (1.28%) (MANNA E TOLEDO, 2008).

Table 1 lists the bird species, as well as their popular names and migratory *status*.

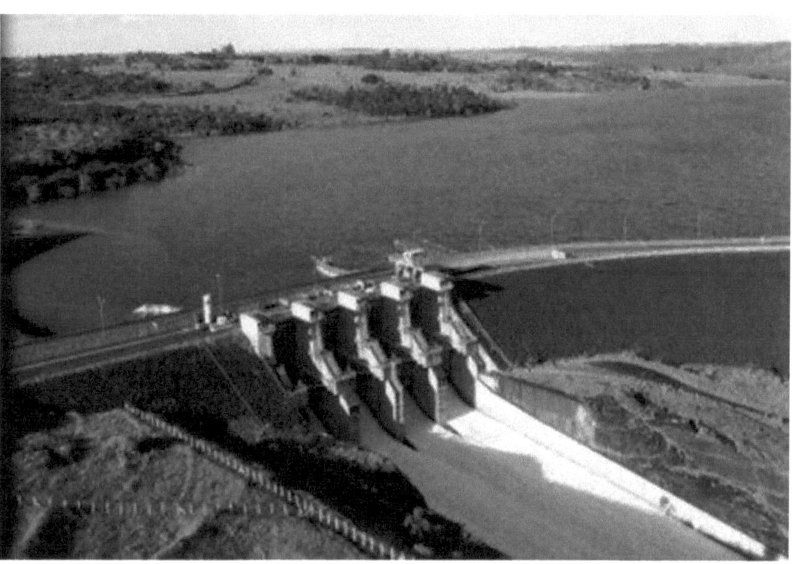

Figure 6 - Amador Aguiar I hydroelectric plant. Source: CCBE (2009).

The impacts arising from the construction of a hydroelectric plant are divided into positive and negative, whose magnitude is related to the size, volume, retention time of the reservoir, geographical location and part of the river involved (ZANZARINI; COSTA, 2008). The Amador Aguiar I and II hydroelectric dam complex covers a directly affected area of 6,400 ha, including land in the municipalities of Indianópolis, Uberlândia and Araguari. HPP Amador Aguiar I has an installed capacity of 240 MW, occupying an area of 18 km^2 and HPP Amador Aguiar II produces 210 MW, occupying an area of 46 km2 (CCBE, 2009).

Hydroelectric dams can cause changes in the avifauna of the area affected by their reservoir, such as the attraction of some aquatic birds, including species originating from North America (SICK, 1983).

Some poultry farms (chickens, hens and turkeys) are close to the Amador Aguiar I and II hydroelectric dams (Figure 8). Table 13 shows 39 properties within 1,000 m of the dam's edge, with a flock of just over 111,000 birds housed in this area, including free-range and industrial poultry. It should be noted that migratory birds from North America have been identified in the area surrounding the reservoir.

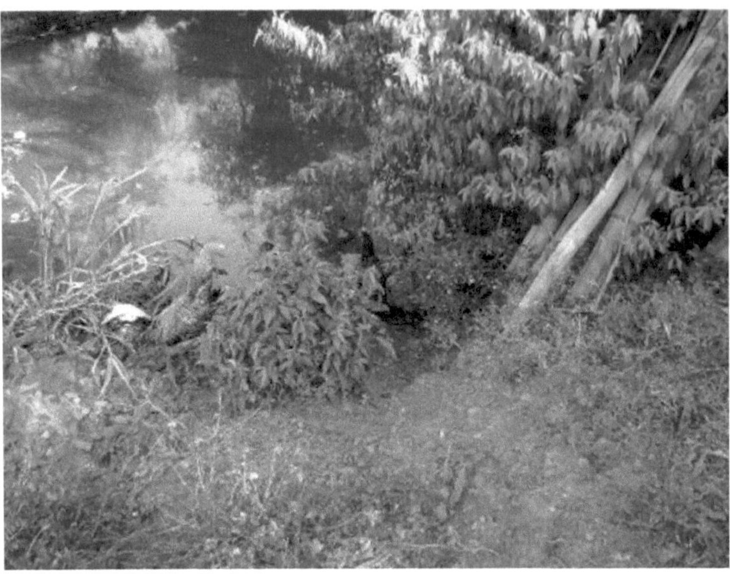

Figure 7 - Raising free-range poultry on the banks of the Amador Aguiar I hydroelectric power station.

Source: REZENDE (2009).

Table 13

Distance of poultry farms from the shore of the Amador Aguiar I and II Hydroelectric Power Plants.

Distance (m)	Industrial Creation	No. of birds	Caipira breeding	No. of birds
0 - 200	1	50.000	5	195
201 - 500	02	53.500	12	895
501-1000	01	3.600	18	3.341
Total	04	107.100	35	4.431

Source: Rural survey, 2006.

Adapted from REZENDE (2009).

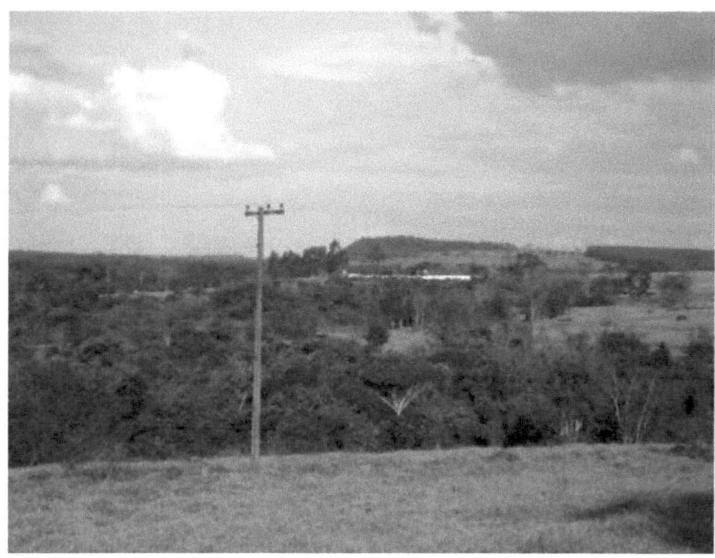

Figure 8 - Industrial broiler farm located less than 1,000 m from the edge of the Amador Aguiar I hydroelectric power station dam.

Source: REZENDE (2009).

The four migratory species found in the avifauna survey of the Amador Aguiar I and II Hydroelectric Power Plant area are described below.

Solitary* sandpiper *(Tringa solitaria)

It measures around 18 cm (Figure 9). It is considered to be a solitary visitor, occurring in all regions of Brazil; it lives by the water's edge, including trees and flooded excavations, a place little sought after by other sandpipers. Its morphology shows the upper side of the wing in a uniform black color, with the habit of swinging the anterior body upwards (SICK, 1983).

In the northern hemisphere, the sandpiper's natural habitat is coniferous forests near lakes (Figure 10). These places are usually sparsely inhabited by other birds. In winter it is found on the muddy banks of small ponds, rivers and marshes. Approximately 90% of the world's Sandpiper population is located in the Boreal Forest of North America, from western Alaska to Labrador and from south to north along the shores of the Great Lakes. Breeding pairs are established in May, producing three to five eggs incubated by the male and female. The sandpiper crosses the entire southern tip of the United States, moving along the east coast of the Rocky Mountains, towards Central America, the Caribbean and South America, reaching as far as eastern Argentina (Figure 11). Unlike other birds, they migrate in small flocks. This species is essentially insectivorous (mainly mosquitoes and small larvae), supplementing its diet with small crustaceans, molluscs, worms, fish, ras and tadpoles (BOREAL BIRDS, 2009).

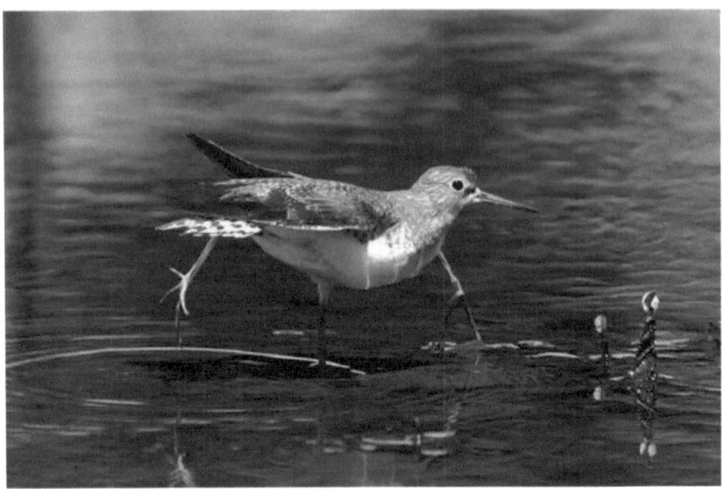

Figure 9 - Detail showing the sandpiper. Source: BOREAL BIRDS (2009).

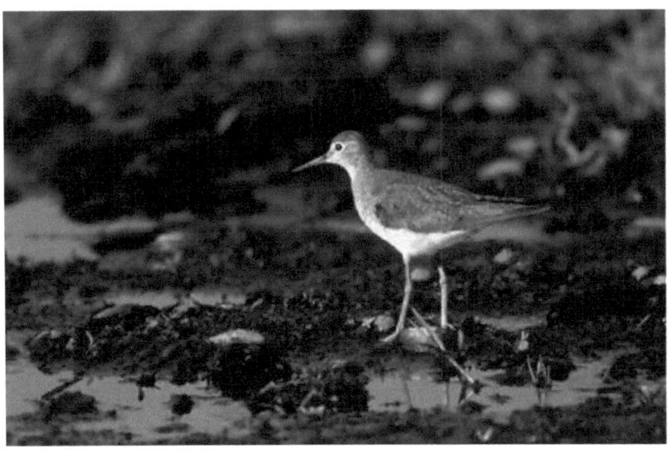

Figure 10 - Sandpiper in its natural habitat.

Source: BOREAL BIRDS (2009).

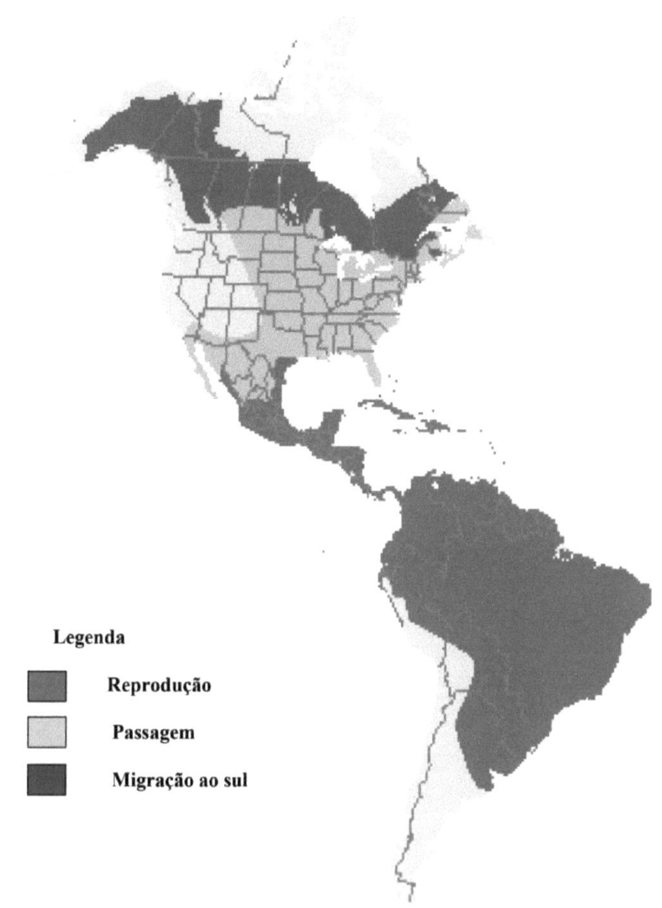

Figure 11 - Sandpiper migration on the American continent.

Source: CORNELL LAB OF ORNITHOLOGY (2009).

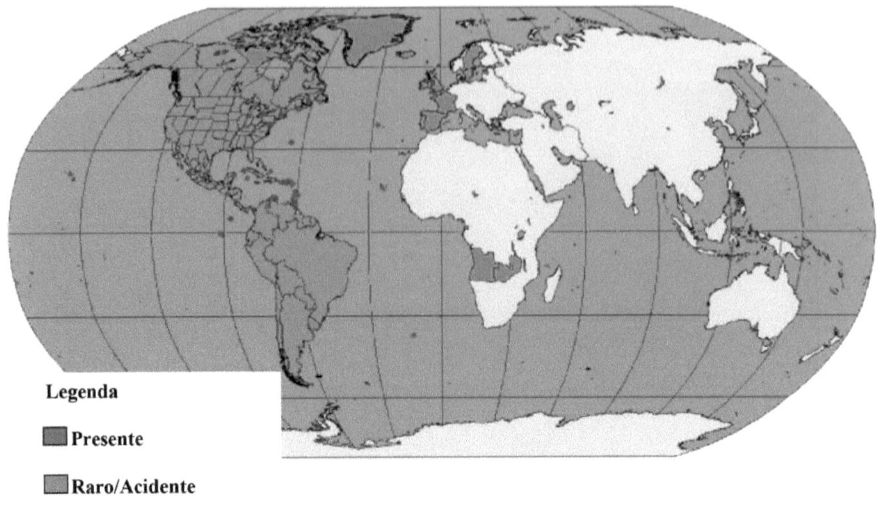

Figure 12 - Distribution of the Solitary Sandpiper around the world Source: AVIBASE (2009).

Spotted Sandpiper (*Actitis macularius*)

It is around 19 cm long, slender and has a white line on the upper side of its wings and a black underside with a white area in the middle. It lives on the stony and muddy banks of rivers, almost always among the vegetation (Figure 13). It frequents mangroves, where it perches on roots and branches to spend the night. It occurs in most of Brazil; in the Amazon it is very active in September, showing reproductive plumage and emitting sound signals. The genus *Actitis* can be included in the genus *Tringa* (SICK, 1983).

It is estimated that 73% of the population is present in the Boreal Forest of the northern hemisphere. It inhabits lake areas, streams and riverbeds, both inland and along the coast (Figure 14). Nests are found from the northern portion of Alaska and Canada to the southern United States, with around four eggs in each nest (BOREAL BIRDS, 2009).

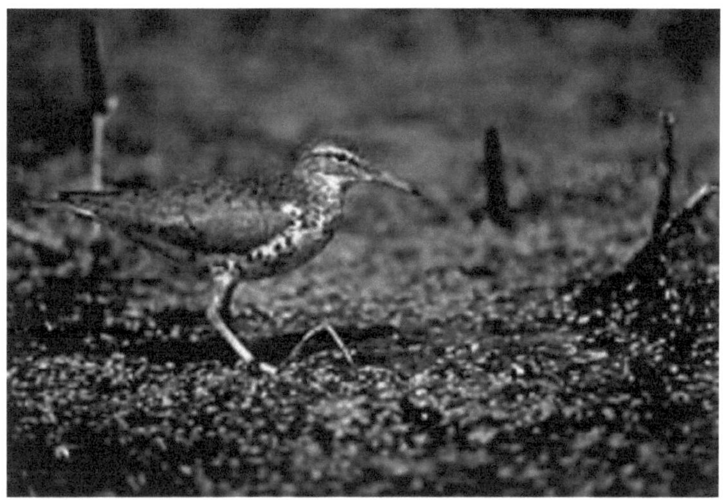

Figure 13 - Spotted sandpiper in its natural habitat.

Source: BOREAL BIRDS (2009).

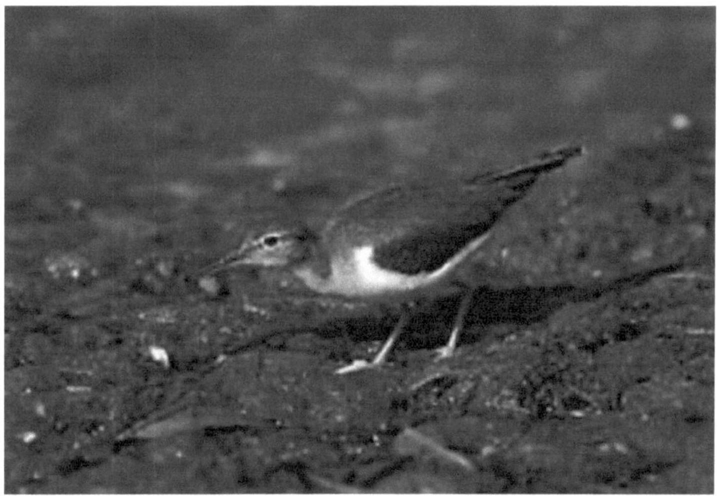

Figure 14 - Detail showing the painted curlew.

Source: BOREALBIRDS (2009).

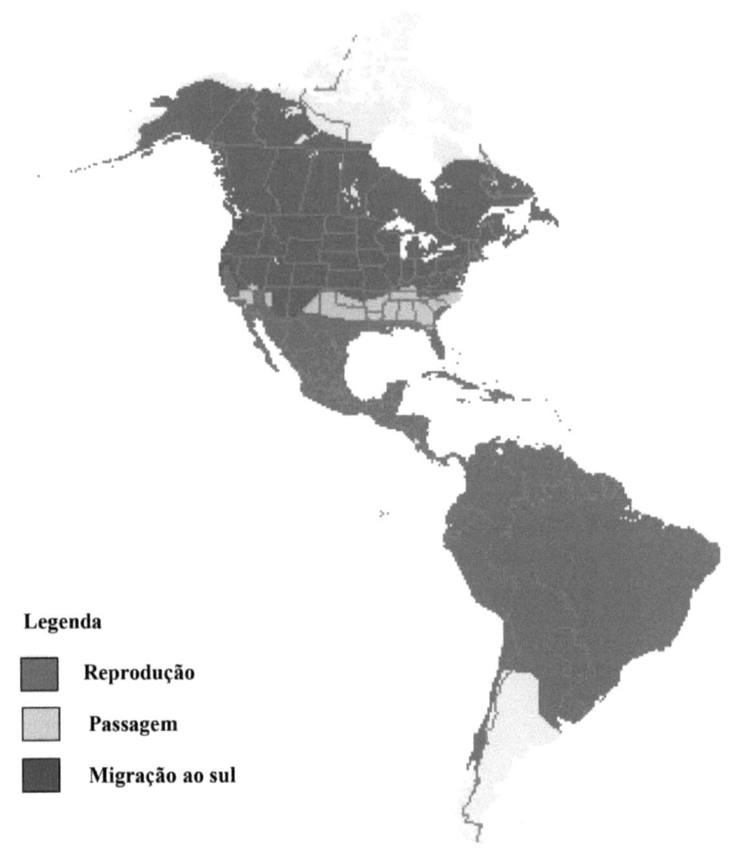

Figura 15 - Migration of the Spotted Sandpiper on the American continent.

Source: CORNELL LAB OF ORNITHOLOGY (2009).

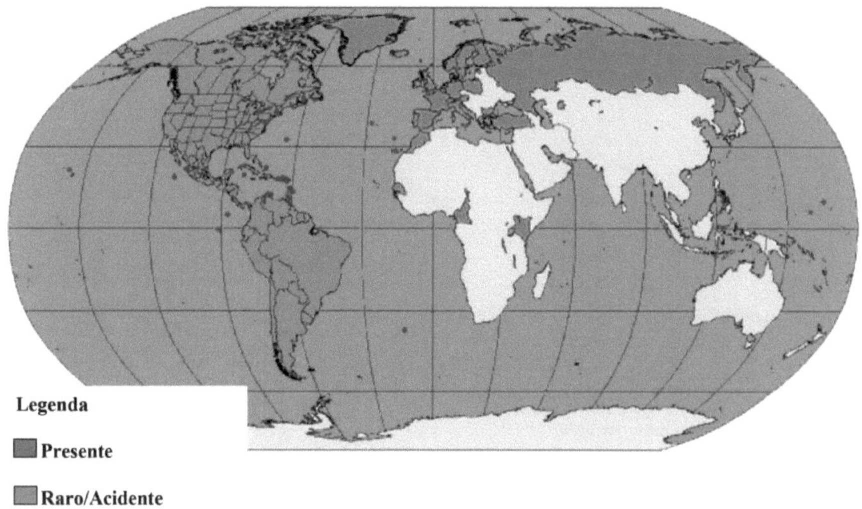

Figura 16 - Distribution of the Spotted Sandpiper around the world. Source: AVIBASE, 2009.

Banded swallow (*Hirundo rustica*)

Approximately 15.5 cm long, it migrates from the Northern Hemisphere. Its characteristic feature is its long tail, deeply notched and crossed by a white band (not visible from above when the tail is closed). The immature individual has a much shorter tail and a pale rusty underside, with a whitish forehead and abdomen (see Figure 17). The Band-rumped Swallow lives in the countryside, in marshes, on farms and in areas close to humans. They occur periodically throughout Brazil, sometimes appearing in hundreds to thousands between September and March; in October they are common in Amapà and in November in Rio de Janeiro. Their migrations extend as far as Tierra del Fuego (SICK, 1983).

It is estimated that the barn swallow represents 8% of the bird species found in the Boreal Forest of the American continent during the breeding phase. It inhabits farmland, suburban areas, swamps and riverbanks (Figure 18). The nests contain four to six eggs. Its diet is basically made up of insects: flies, grasshoppers, crickets, dragonflies and others. The barn swallow migrates long distances (up to 8,700 km), occurring from the north of America, as far as Alaska, through the south of the United States and northern Mexico to the south of Argentina (Figure 19). Normally, during migration, they travel during the day, taking their meals during the journey. This species is light and fast, and can travel up to 375 km a day. Determining the true whereabouts of any population of barn swallows during migration is complicated because, during their movements, they join other flocks that are also migrating (BOREAL BIRDS, 2009).

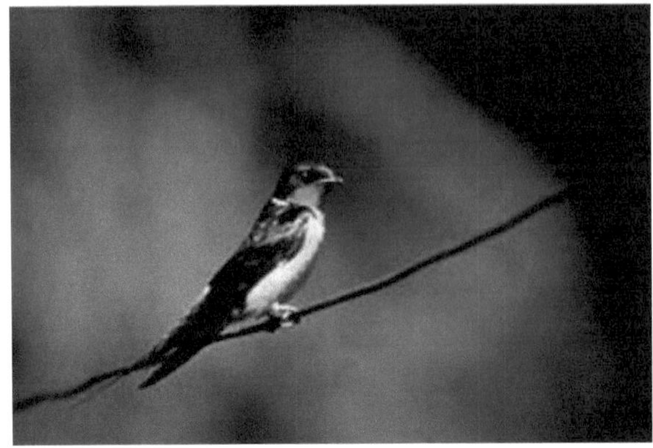

Figure 17 - Detail of the barn swallow.

Source: BOREAL BIRDS (2009).

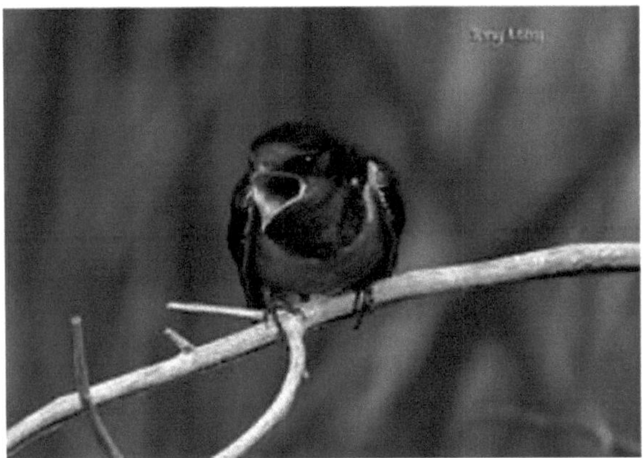

Figure 18 - Banded swallow emitting a sound signal.

Source: AVIBASE (2009).

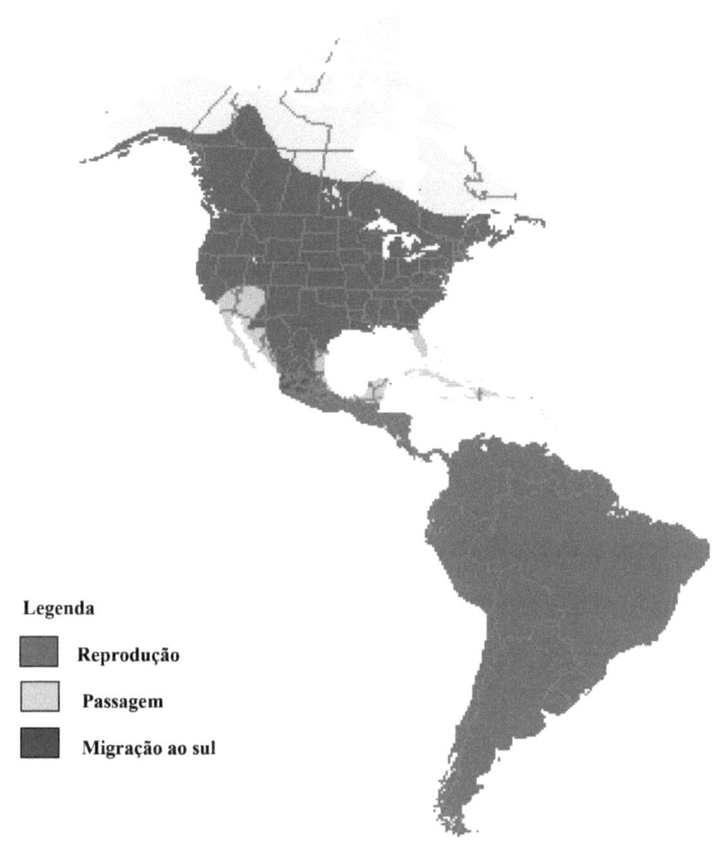

Figure 19 - Swallow migration on the American continent.

Source: CORNELL LAB OF ORNITHOLOGY (2009).

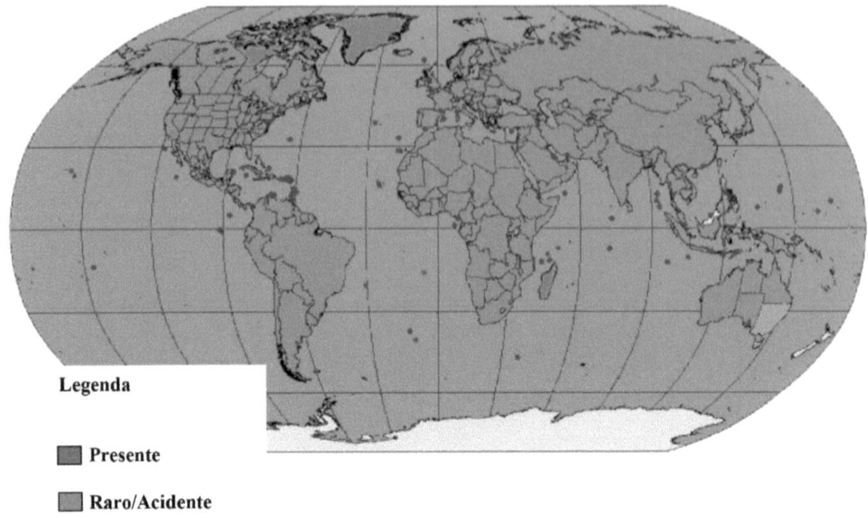

Figure 20 - Distribution of the barn swallow in the world. Source: AVIBASE (2009).

Ring-billed Swallow (*Petrochelidon pyrrhonota*)

Measuring approximately 14.3 cm, it is a northern migrant, a robust species with a relatively short tail and a complicated design: whitish forehead, bright blue cap, brown anterior throat and nuchal band, ferruginous uropygium. It ranges from North America to Argentina. It inhabits the countryside, always in flocks, with occurrences in various parts of Brazil (Amazonas - November -, Sao Paulo (January to March), Santa Catarina (January), Rio Grande do Sul (March). Several ringed individuals from New York have been captured in the states of Sao Paulo and Santa Catarina (SICK, 1983).

It is estimated that 12% of North American species are located in the Boreal Forest during the breeding season (Figure 21). They live in rocky places, in swamps and on river banks (Figure 22). Nests are made in colonies, with four to six eggs in each. The introduction of sparrows into their habitats has been a disaster for these birds, as they usurp their nests and make the swallows abandon their colonies. Migration normally takes place in two groups: one moving down the eastern slope of the American continent and the other along the Mississippi River valley, towards South America (Figure 23) (BOREAL BIRDS, 2009).

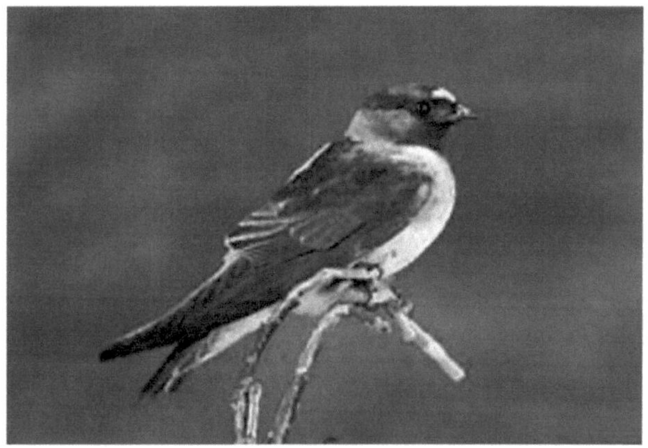

Figure 21 - Ring-billed Swallow in its natural habitat.

Source: BOREAL BIRDS (2009).

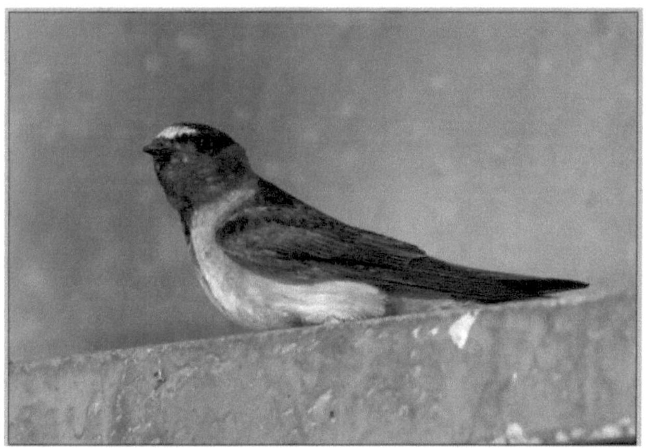

Figure 22 - Detail of the ring-billed swallow

Figure: BOREAL BIRDS (2009).

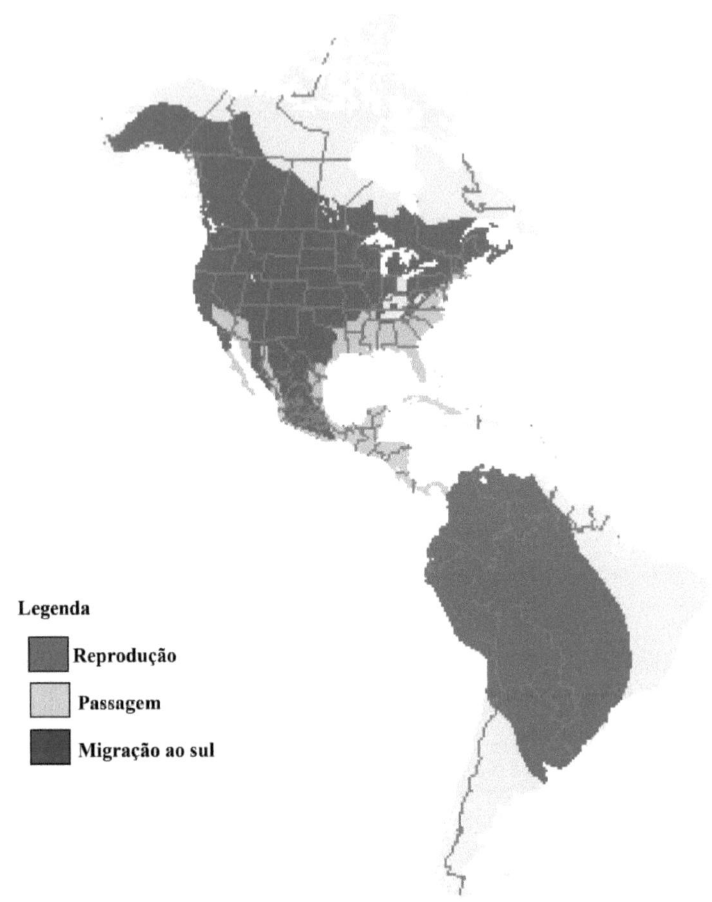

Figure 23 - Migration of the Ring-billed Swallow on the American continent.

Source: CORNELL LAB OF ORNITHOLOGY (2009).

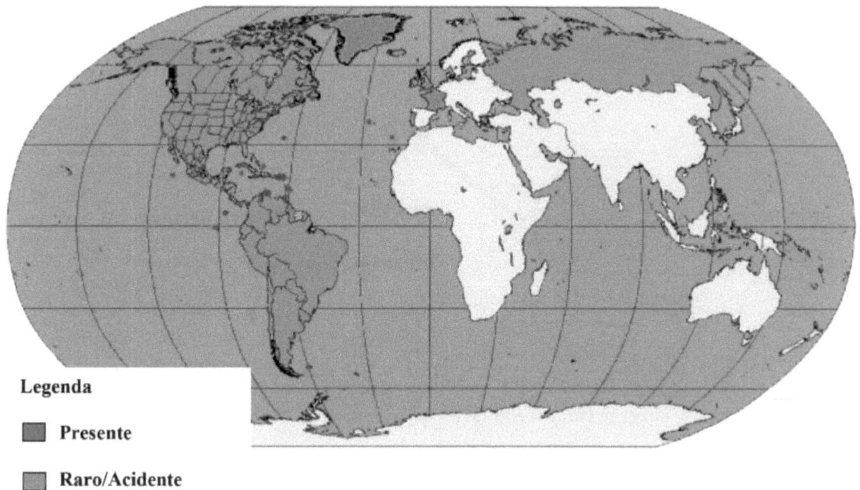

Figure 24 - Distribution of the Ring-billed Swallow around the world. Source: AVIBASE (2009).

3.5 Avian Influenza

Avian influenza is an infectious disease caused by the type A influenza virus, which belongs to the Orthomyxoviridae family and is a negative-sense, enveloped, single-stranded RNA virus with a viral genome made up of eight segments and 10 viral proteins. It has two glycoproteins on its outer surface: hemagglutinin (HA) and neuraminidase (NA) (Figure 25). Influenza A subtypes have 16 types of hemagglutinins and nine types of neuraminidases. These proteins, which have antigenic characteristics, are responsible for classifying the virus subtype. For example, H5N1 is the subtype that contains 5 types of hemagglutinin and 1 type of neuraminidase (CAPUA; ALEXANDER, 2009).

The avian influenza virus can cause infections in birds with clinical symptoms of low pathogenicity, known as Low Pathogenic Avian Influenza Virus (LPAI) or with clinical symptoms of high pathogenicity, known as High Pathogenic Avian Influenza Virus (HPAI).

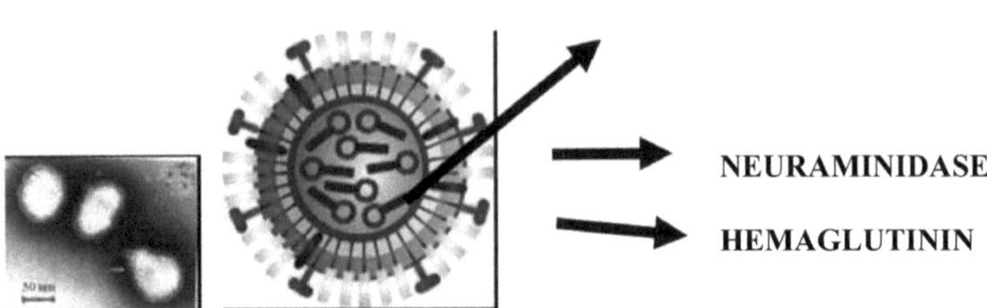

Source: WEBSTER et al. (1992).

Of the subtypes found, only the H5, H7 and H10 viruses caused IAAP in susceptible species, although not all individuals from these groups are virulent (CAPUA and ALEXANDER, 2009).

The avian influenza virus is capable of infecting a wide variety of birds, including free-living birds, captured and caged birds, domestic ducks, chickens, turkeys and other domestic birds (CAPUA; ALEXANDER, 2009).

Systematic research into influenza in wild birds began to be considered in the mid-1970s. These investigations revealed that wild birds, especially aquatic birds, are natural reservoirs for a large number of influenza viruses. The main representatives are species from the Anatidae, Charadriiformes and Passariformes families (CAPUA; ALEXANDER, 2009).

In addition to avian species, Influenza A viruses affect other animals, including humans, pigs, horses and marine mammals (WEBSTER et al., 1992).

Wild waterfowl are natural hosts of the disease and have probably carried it for years (Figure 26). It is known that these birds can harbor influenza viruses, but mostly in their low pathogenic form. Evidence has shown that migratory birds may be responsible for introducing LPAI viruses into commercial poultry farms, which then mutate into strains of IAAP-causing viruses and eventually cause infection in the human population (CAPUA; ALEXANDER, 2009).

Wild bird species, especially waterfowl such as ducks and teals, harbor IAAP and IABP viruses, without the obligatory presentation of clinical symptoms. Contact between domestic and migratory birds has been the source of many epidemic outbreaks. Avian influenza (AI) can occasionally be spread to the human and animal population following direct contact between people and infected birds (WEBSTER et al., 1992).

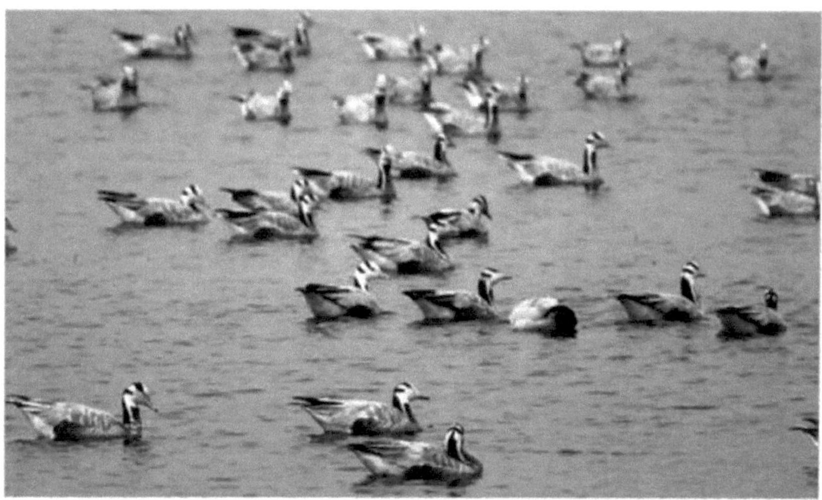

Figure 26 - Migratory waterfowl.

Source: REUTERS (2009).

The LPAI viruses cause mild symptoms in birds, which can go unnoticed. The highly pathogenic forms of LPAI are more marked when it comes to observing symptoms in birds: severe depression, inappetence, facial edema with swollen and purplish crest and dewlap, difficulty breathing with nasal discharge, a severe drop in egg laying, a decrease in water and feed consumption of 20% or more and sudden death, which can reach 100% of the flock within 48 hours. Of the subtypes found, only the H5, H7 and H10 viruses caused IAAP in susceptible species, although not all individuals in these groups are virulent. Of these, H5N1 and H7N7 were the most frequently isolated subtypes in outbreaks of the disease. The H5N1 subtype is largely responsible for the sacrifice and death of millions of birds in Asia, and is considered endemic in many countries on this continent (Figure 27) (CAPUA; ALEXANDER, 2009).

The spread of H5N1 in the poultry population can pose risks to the human population. The risk refers to direct infection, when the agent passes from birds to the human population, resulting in a very severe disease. Of the cases that have occurred in the world, the H5N1 virus has been the main culprit, especially in Asia, with a high mortality rate (TOLLIS; DI TRANI, 2002).

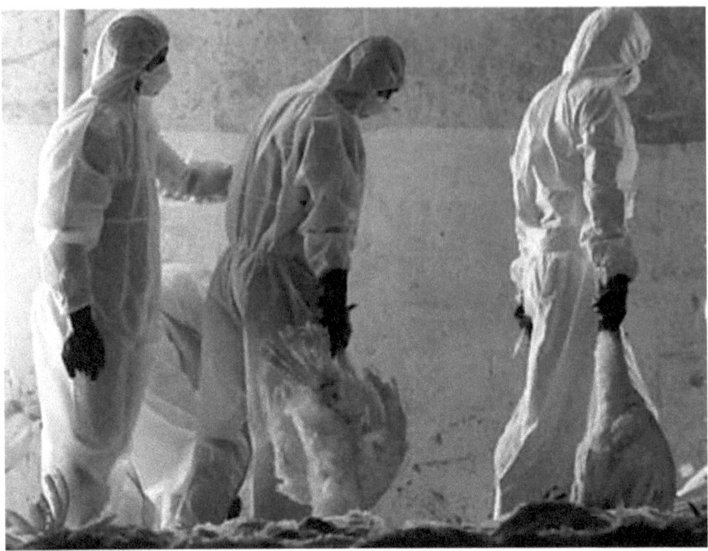

Figure 27 - Destruction of birds affected by avian influenza.

Source: REUTERS (2009).

In human H5N1 infections, unlike seasonal influenza, in which infections cause only mild respiratory symptoms, the patient's clinical condition worsens rapidly, with a high mortality rate. Primary viral pneumonia with an unfavorable course, evolving into systemic failure, is common (Figure 26). Most cases occurred in healthy children and young people. These cases were characterized by the presence of highly pathogenic subtypes, due to direct contact with infected birds. In 1997 there was the first detection of bird-to-human transmission of the H5N1 strain, during an outbreak in Hong Kong. The virus caused severe respiratory illness in 18 people, with six deaths. Since then, other cases of H5N1 have occurred in the human population (VRANJAC, 2006).

The virus is spread between birds through saliva, nasal secretions and feces. Spread to susceptible birds occurs when they come into contact with contaminated droppings. Human cases of H5N1 are the result of contact with infected birds or fomites (VRANJAC, 2006).

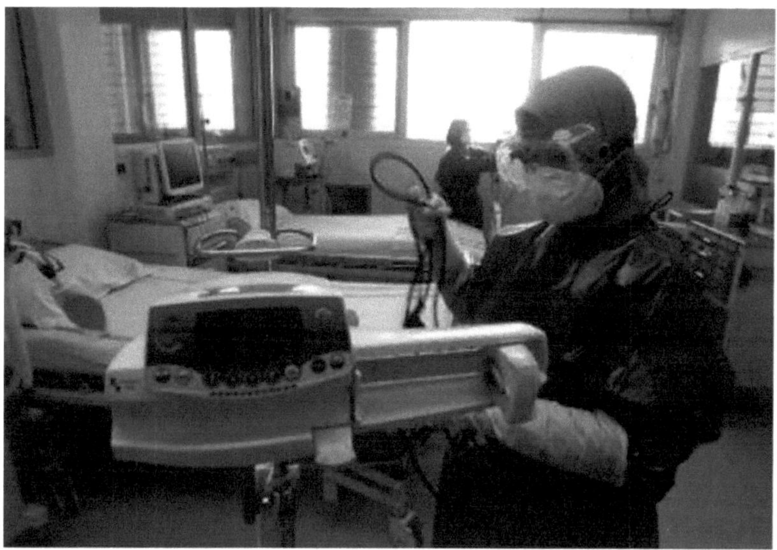

Figure 28 - Isolation for influenza victims.

Source: REUTERS (2009).

There are still no scientific studies proving the transmission of the virus between humans, although the focus of attention is on the possibility of genetic mutation of the circulating virus, especially in Southeast Asia, leading to the transformation of the AI virus into a new variant, capable of being transmitted between humans. In this sense, the threat becomes greater with the possibility of a combination with the H1N1 subtype, responsible for influenza A, capable of being transmitted from one person to another. This change could lead to a pandemic situation, which, according to the WHO, assuming the most favorable scenario, could cause between two million and 7.4 million deaths worldwide (KHALAKDINA; NARAIN, 2005).

In Asia, the close coexistence of humans with domestic birds, especially ducks and geese, may have facilitated the occurrence of human cases in the countries of this continent (Figure 29) (WHO, 2007).

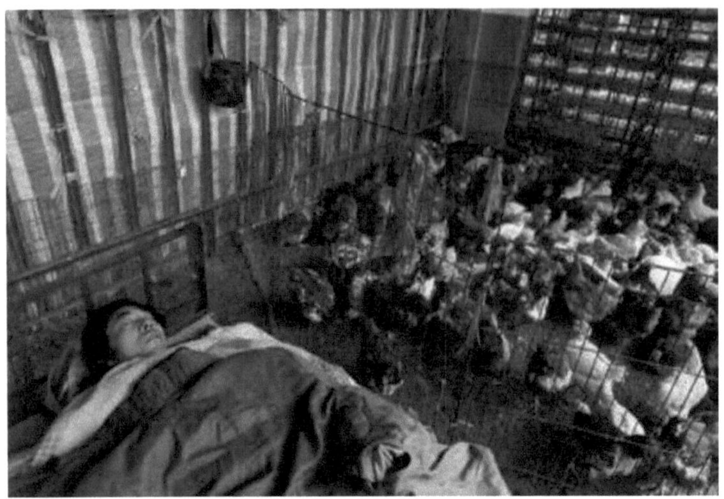

Figure 29 - Detail of the close coexistence of man and bird.

Source: REUTERS (2009).

3.5.1 The siege in the world

Since December 2003, some Asian countries have reported outbreaks of IAAP in chickens and ducks: Afghanistan, Saudi Arabia, Azerbaijan, Bangladesh, Cambodia, China, South Korea, Hong Kong, India, Indonesia, Iraq, Israel, Japan, Jordan, Kazakhstan, Kuwait, Laos, Malaysia, Myanmar, Nepal, Palestine, Pakistan, Taiwan, Thailand and Vietnam. Subsequently, the AI virus spread to the West and caused alarm about the imminence of an influenza pandemic. Outbreaks of birds contaminated by the H5N1 virus, which causes the disease, have been detected in Albania, Austria, Denmark, France, Germany, Greece, Hungary, Italy, Poland, the Czech Republic, Romania, Russia, Serbia and Montenegro, Sweden, Switzerland, Turkey and Ukraine. Some African countries, such as Benin, Burkina Faso, Cameroon, Côte d'Ivoire, Djibouti, Egypt, Ghana, Nigeria, Sudan and Togo have also presented the problem. The spread of IAAP, with outbreaks occurring in several countries at the same time, is historically unprecedented and of great concern for human and animal health. Of particular concern in terms of risks to human health is the detection of the IAAP virus known as FLU A/H5N1 as the cause of most of these outbreaks (OIE, 2009b).

As of November 27, 2009, the WHO (United Nations Organization) has confirmed a total of 444 cases of people infected with the H5N1 virus in Azerbaijan, Bangladesh, Cambodia, China, Djibouti, Egypt, Indonesia, Iraq, Laos, Myanmar, Nigeria, Pakistan, Vietnam, Thailand, Turkey and Vietnam, leading to 262 deaths since 2003 (see Figure 30) (WHO, 2009).

3.5.2 Avian Influenza Outbreaks in North America

In Canada, the first reports of AI outbreaks in domestic poultry occurred in the 60s. In 1966, the IAAP virus (A/turkey/Ontario/7732/1966 (H5N9)) was isolated in breeding turkeys. From then until 2004, the isolated viruses corresponded to the IABP viruses, such as H5N9 in 1967, H5N2 in 1968 (PASICK; BERHANE; MACGREVY, 2009).

In the 1980s, several subtypes were isolated from turkey farms, including H5, H6, H7 and H9 subtypes. In the 1990s, out of a total of 24 isolations of the AI virus, 12 originated from turkey farming, six from chicken farming, five from domestic duck farming and one from quail farming. The subtypes found in turkey farming were H3N2, H6N1, H6N2, H6N8 and H7N1, which are of low pathogenicity. In the case of broiler chickens, the H1N1, H6N8, H7N3 and H10N7 subtypes of low pathogenicity and two H7N3 subtypes of high pathogenicity were isolated. In domestic duck farming, the IABP viruses H2N5, H3N2, H4N6, H5N2 and H11N9 have been isolated (PASICK; BERHANE; MACGREVY, 2009).

In 2000, a flock of breeding turkeys in the state of Ontario showed high mortality and egg production problems as a result of infection with an IAPB H7N1 virus (CAPUA and ALEXANDER, 2009).

In 2004, Canada notified the first case of IAAP to the OIE. The outbreak occurred on a broiler farm in British Columbia, due to a mildly pathogenic H7N3 strain that underwent a rapid virulence transformation, behaving like an IAAP virus (OIE, 2009 b). There was a depopulation of 17 million birds in the entire control area, with an estimated loss of 380 million Canadian dollars. In 2005, the H5N2 subtype was isolated from a commercial domestic duck farm in British Columbia. The same subtype had been isolated with a high prevalence in wild ducks found on lakes, 120 km from the commercial farm. In 2007, the

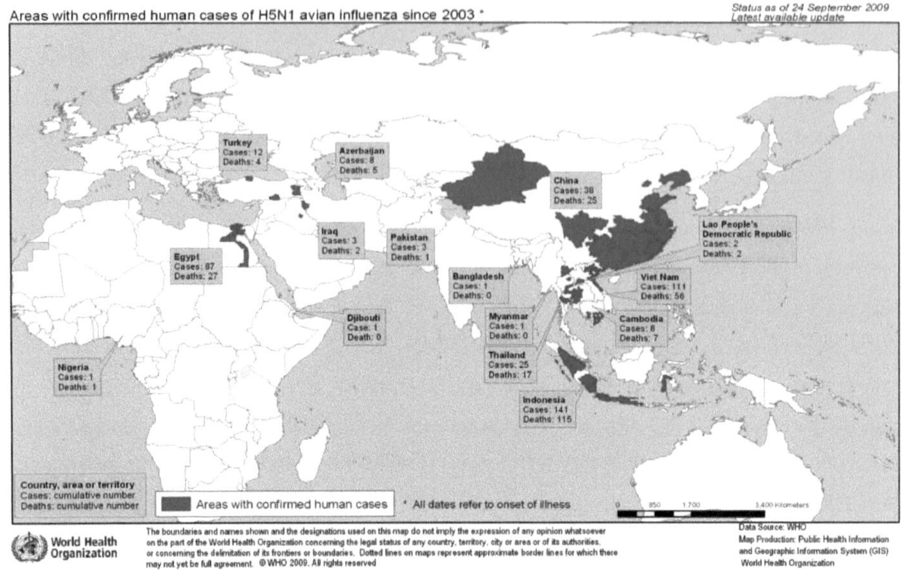

Figura 30 - Countries with human cases of H5N1 avian influenza from 2003 to 24/09/2009.

Source: WHO (2009).

IAAP H7N3 subtype in Saskatchewan, in a region of low poultry density. Phylogenetic analysis of this subtype showed a high degree of identity with other subtypes isolated from wild waterfowl in 2006 and 2007 in North America (PASICK; BERHANE; MACGREVY, 2009).

In 2000, a flock of breeding turkeys in the state of Ontario showed high mortality and egg production problems as a result of infection with an IAPB H7N1 virus (CAPUA; ALEXANDER, 2009).

In 2004, Canada notified the first case of IAAP to the OIE. The outbreak occurred on a broiler farm in British Columbia, due to a mildly pathogenic H7N3 strain that underwent a rapid virulence transformation, behaving like an IAAP virus (OIE, 2009). There was a depopulation of 17 million birds in the entire control area, with an estimated loss of 380 million Canadian dollars. In 2005, the H5N2 subtype was isolated from a commercial domestic duck farm in British Columbia. The same subtype had been isolated with a high prevalence in wild ducks found on lakes, 120 km from the commercial farm. In 2007, the IAAP H7N3 subtype was isolated in Saskatchewan, in a region of low poultry density. Phylogenetic analysis of this subtype showed a high degree of identity with other subtypes isolated from wild waterfowl in 2006 and 2007 in North America (PASICK; BERHANE; MACGREVY, 2009).

In 2005, the National Wild Bird Monitoring Program was introduced in Canada and, in the first year of research, 37% of the materials analyzed were positive for the AI virus, 5% of which were of the

H5 subtype, with two H5N1 samples. In 2006, with the introduction of research on dead birds, the possible incursion of the H5N1 subtype of Eurasian origin was admitted. In 2007, the H7 subtype was found for the first time. In these three years of research, all the hemagglutinin subtypes have been identified, except for H14 and H15, and all the neuraminidase subtypes, from N1 to N9 (PASICK; BERHANE; MACGREVY, 2009).

The first reported outbreak of AI in the United States occurred in 1924 and 1925, affecting nine states. The first signs of the disease were a high mortality rate of unknown cause in the New York chicken markets. Later, the disease appeared in the chicken markets of Pennsylvania and New Jersey. This outbreak produced an economic impact estimated at one million dollars, with the death and elimination of 600,000 birds.

The disease then spread to the markets of Connecticut, Illinois, Indiana, Michigan, Missouri and West Virginia. The main way the disease spread was through the transportation of live birds by train. The outbreak was controlled by adopting quarantine measures, depopulation and hygiene procedures. In May 1929 there was a small outbreak in New Jersey, affecting four flocks of birds, which was controlled in August 1929 (HALVORSON, 2009).

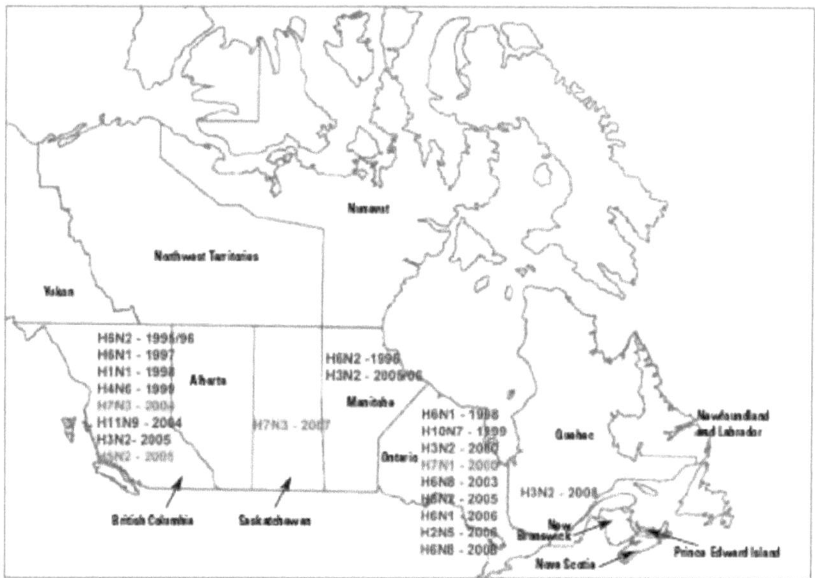

Figura 31 - Geographical distribution of Avian Influenza viruses in poultry in Canada from 1998 to 2008.

Source: PASICK; BERHANE; MACGREVY (2009).

From the 1960s onwards, small outbreaks of LPAI were identified through virus isolation or serological tests. From the mid-1970s to the present day, nine large-scale outbreaks of LPAI have been identified in the USA (HALVORSON, 2009).

There have been four outbreaks of LPAI in Minnesota. In 1978 there was an outbreak involving the commercial rearing of two million turkeys, 24,000 breeding turkeys and 165,000 egg-producing hens, generating a loss in direct costs of 16 million dollars. The subtypes isolated were H4N8, H6N1, H6N2, H6N8 and H9N2. In 1988, a new outbreak of LPAI involved 258 batches of turkeys and one batch of broiler breeders, with an estimated loss of 5.8 million dollars. The subtypes H2N2, H4N6, H5N6, H7N9, H8N4 and H9N2 were identified. In 1991 the outbreak involved 110 flocks of turkeys with influenza subtypes H1, H4, H5, H6 and H7. Economic losses were estimated at 1.5 million dollars. In 1995, the outbreak involved 178 flocks of turkeys, infected mainly with the H9N2 subtype and also with the H1N1, H6N8 and H10N7 subtypes. The damage was estimated at 8.2 million dollars. All AI outbreaks in Minnesota have been associated with wild birds, mainly due to their contact with free-range turkeys (HALVORSON, 2009).

In April 1983, an H5N2 subtype of LPAI was detected in Pennsylvania. In October of the same year, a flock of laying hens showed severe clinical signs with a drop in production and 89% mortality. The virus isolated was also H5N2. This was the first documented case of virulence reversal from an IABP virus to an IAAP virus. With the decision to eliminate all H5N2-positive flocks, 17 million birds were destroyed in 448 flocks in Pennsylvania, Virginia and New Jersey, with an economic impact of 156 million dollars (HALVORSON, 2009).

A new outbreak of H5N2 appeared in 1986, initially affecting the state of Pennsylvania and then New York, Massachusetts and Ohio. This outbreak was controlled through the adoption of sanitary measures, including the destruction of infected birds, quarantine and health education. An epidemiological investigation directly correlated the contamination of poultry farms with the crates used to transport live birds to market. Molecular research later showed that it was the same virus responsible for the 1983/1984 outbreak (HALVORSON, 2009).

In April 1995, an outbreak of AI began in Utah in free-living turkey farms, with isolation of the H7N3 subtype. The origin of the infection was associated with contact with wild birds. Economic losses were estimated at 2.7 million dollars (HALVORSON, 2009).

Pennsylvania again had a case of AI, this time of LPAI in December 1996, involving more than 2.6 million birds in 47 flocks, with egg-producing hens being the most affected. The origin of the outbreak was associated with live birds sold on the market, with isolation of the H7N2 subtype. Losses were estimated at six million dollars (HALVORSON, 2009).

In February 2000, the H6N2 subtype was isolated from backyard poultry and in a flock of commercial egg producers, with probable evidence of the involvement of wild birds. In 2001, the H6N2 subtype continued to be isolated and in 2002 involved 37 commercial egg production flocks, at least 43 chicken farms, nine turkey farms, two chicken breeding farms and one turkey breeding farm. More than 20 million birds were affected, making it the largest LPAI outbreak in terms of number of birds. The direct and indirect costs were estimated at 40 million dollars (HALVORSON, 2009).

In March 2002, the H7N2 subtype was isolated in Virginia after the appearance of respiratory signs and a drop in egg production in turkey breeders. 197 flocks were affected and 4.7 million birds were destroyed, at a total cost of 166 million dollars (HALVORSON, 2009).

In February 2003, in the state of Conneticut, there was an outbreak of LPAI H7N2 in four farms, compromising 3.5 million commercial egg producers and an economic loss that exceeded 30 million dollars (HALVORSON, 2009).

In 2004, an outbreak was identified in a small chicken farm in Texas, involving H5N2. The birds from this farm were returning from a live bird market. The molecular study showed that it was the IAAP A/chicken/Scotland/1959 sample (HALVORSON, 2009).

In the last three years, new cases of AI involving the H5 and H7 subtypes have been reported to the OIE, with two occurrences in Canada and six in the USA. Approximately 400,000 birds have been directly affected, including chickens, turkeys and game birds. The epidemiological studies showed an unknown origin or cause or the involvement of wild birds (Table 14) (OIE, 2009a).

Table 14

Occurrences of Avian Influenza - Subtypes H5 and H7 - in the USA and Canada from 2007 to 2009

Year	Parents	State	Cepa	Animal Species	Origin or Suspicion	Birds affected
2007	USA	Virginia	H5N2	Turkeys	Unknown	25.600
2007	USA	Virginia	H5N1	Turkeys	Unknown	54.000
2007	USA	Nebraska	H7N9	Turkeys	Unknown	144.000
2007	Canada	Saskatchewan	H7N3	Chicken Chicken	Wild birds	49.100
2008	USA	Arkansas	H7N3	Game birds	Unknown	16.000
2008	USA	Idaho	H5N8	Turkeys	Wild animals	30.000
2009	Canada	British Columbia	Under study	Chicken	Unknown	57.309
2009	USA	Kentucky	H7N9		Unknown	20.000

Source: OIE , 2009a.

Adapted from REZENDE (2009).

3.5.3 The siege in Brazil

The disease is considered exotic in Brazil. The country has had a National Poultry Health Program (PNSA) since 1994 and is constantly monitoring poultry diseases. Continuous surveillance and rapid initial detection of LPAI virus in industrial, subsistence and migratory birds is a factor in preventing the occurrence of highly pathogenic forms of the disease in poultry (BRASIL, 2006).

Active Surveillance, which consists of an epidemiological survey of migratory, free-range and industrial birds, is carried out based on criteria that define the areas classified as being at risk, taking into account the occurrence of the type of migratory bird, the migratory area or site and the human concentration with bird breeding (Table 15). The migratory site corresponds to the roosting areas that the birds use to feed and rest on their way to and from their migratory journeys.

The epidemiological surveys carried out in 2005 and 2006 covering specific monitoring sites in the states of Rio Grande do Sul, Bahia, Para and Pernambuco recorded the occurrence of the low pathogenic avian influenza virus (LPAI), with the H3 and H4 subtypes. The survey included the collection of material for analysis from migratory, resident and domestic birds. The work was coordinated by the Ministry of Agriculture, Livestock and Supply (Table 16).

Table 15

Areas of Brazilian territory where active surveillance for avian influenza is carried out.

UF	Municipalities and Regions	Sitio	Criteria[6]
BA	Itaparica Island	Nails	3
BA	Jandaira	Mangue Seco	1,2
BA	New Viçosa	Red Crown	3
BA	Camaçari	CETREL	2,3
MA	Baia de Sâo José: Sâo José Ribamar and others	Panaquatira	2,3
MA	Cururupu	Guara	1,2
MS	Corumba	Pantanal	3
PA	Breves, Sâo Sebastiâo da Boa Vista	Marajó Island	2,3
PA	Vigia and Sâo Caetano de Odivelas	Marajó Bay	2,3
PA	Salinópolis	Salinópolis	2,3
PE	Igarassu	Airplane crown	1,2
PE	Fernando de Noronha	Fernando de Noronha	2
RN	Galinhos	Galinhos	1,2
RS	Rio Grande and Santa Vitória do Palmar	Taim	2,3
RS	Tavares and Mostardas	Fish Lagoon	1,2
SC	Coastal Islands and Ararangua	Ararangua	2,3
SC	Barra Velha and Tijucas	Tijucas	2,3
SP	Coastal Islands and Cananéia	Ilha do Cardoso and Ilha Long	2,3

Source: BRASIL (2006).

Table 16

Results obtained in epidemiological surveys for avian influenza in migratory, resident and domestic non-commercial birds in Brazil.

Year	Species	Virus Isolated	Pathogenicity Characterization	Location
2005	*Gallus gallus*	H4	Non-pathogenic	Lagoa do Peixe (RS)
2005	*Sterna hirundo*	H4	Non-pathogenic	Mangue Seco (BA)

6 1- Areas of migratory waterfowl (Anseriformes and Charadriiformes) with positivity for low pathogenic AI in previous surveys.
2- Areas of wild and/or domestic Anseriformes near wetlands, with a concentration of human population and with bird breeding.
3- Areas of concentration and/or reproduction of migratory aquatic birds in continental areas or within 30 km of the coast, without epidemiological information, associated with the concentration of human population and bird breeding (commercial and subsistence).

2005	*Calidris canutus*	H4	Non-pathogenic	Mangue Seco (BA)
2005	*Charadrius wilsonia*	H4	Non-pathogenic	Mangue Seco (BA)
2006	*Arenaria interpres*	H3	Non-pathogenic	Salina (PA)
2006	*Larus dominicanus*	H3	Non-pathogenic	Salina (PA)
2006	*Calidris pusilla*	H3	Non-pathogenic	Salinas (PA)
2006	*Gallus gallus*	H3	Non-pathogenic	Salinas (PA)
2006	*Gallus gallus*	H3	Non-pathogenic	Salinas (PA)
2006	*Gallus gallus*	H3	Non-pathogenic	Coroa do Aviâo (PE)
2006	*Gallus gallus*	H3	Non-pathogenic	Coroa do Aviâo (PE)

Source: BRASIL (2004).

3.6 The Role of Migratory Birds in the Transmission of Avian Influenza

In the broad sense, the term migration is used to refer to the mass directional movements of a large number of individuals of a given species from one location to another. In the strict sense, it refers to the annual and seasonally repeated movement of a given animal population from its breeding area to its feeding and resting areas at a given time of year, returning to its breeding area (Figure 32) (ALVES, 2007).

The occurrence of migratory cycles is due to the search for seasonally available food and the escape from the extremely cold winters of the terrestrial regions furthest from the equator (ALVES, 2007; ELPHICK, 2007). In these regions, the intensity of daily light has been indicated as a factor that stimulates the birds' reproductive organs, with a consequent increase in the accumulation of fat, which serves as a reserve for long-distance movements (ROWAN, 1930 apud ALVES, 2007). In tropical regions, where there is little variation in the photoperiod compared to temperate regions, other factors such as rainfall and consequently flowering and fruiting can serve as a stimulus for migrations (SICK, 1983).

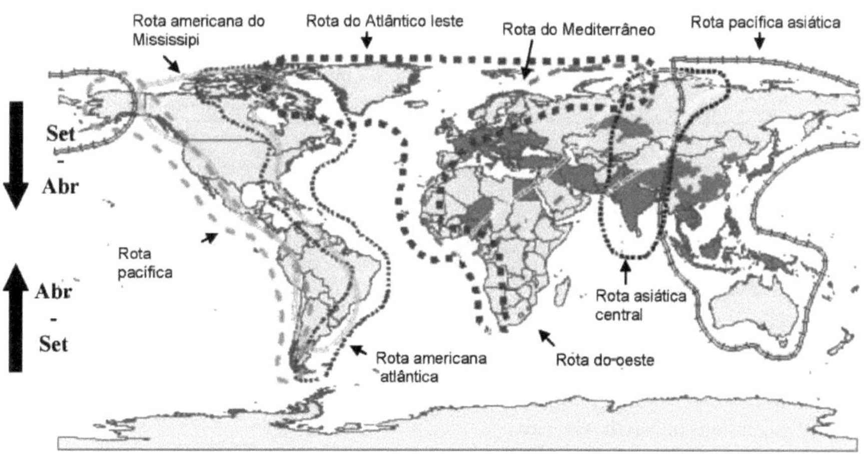

Figure 32 - Main migratory routes of birds in the world. Source: FAO (2009).

The first report of the isolation of the AI virus in wild birds occurred in 1961, in the species *Sterna hirundo*, in South Africa, when an IAAP H5N3 virus caused the death of approximately 1,300 birds (BECKER and UYS, 1988).

Natural AI infections in free-living birds have been described in more than 90 species from 13 taxonomic orders. Many of these species are associated with aquatic habitats and predominantly with two avian orders, the Anseriformes (ducks and geese) and the Charadriiformes (curlews, batuiras) (STALLKNECHT; SHANE, 1988; OLSEN et al., 2006). Belonging to the Anatidae family (order Anseriforme), forty-seven species, out of a total of one hundred and forty-seven ducks and geese, have been linked to AI virus isolates. In the Charadriiform order, isolations have been reported in three families: Scolopacidae, Laridae and Alcidae (STALLKNECHT, 1988).

There is a wide variation in the subtypes of AI viruses among wild bird populations. For ducks, the most common subtypes are H3, H4, H6 and H11 (STALLKNECHT et al., 1990). In cassowaries and curlews, the diversity of subtypes is not so well known, but there are differences between Charadriiformes species compared to ducks (KRAUSS et al., 2004). Nine subtypes of the AI virus occur more frequently in curlews than ducks, including H5, H7, H9 and H13 (KRAUSS et al., 2004).

Studies indicate that the worldwide transmission of the AI virus occurs between two different classes of strains: the Eurasian and the American, the result of a long period of ecological and geographical separation from their hosts. This difference justifies the greater occurrence of the H5N1 subtype in Eurasia than on the American continent. However, the avifauna of North America and Europe and Asia are not completely separate: some birds cross the Bering Strait, simultaneously occupying breeding areas in eastern Russia and northeastern North America. Although the majority of birds from Russia's tundra areas migrate during the winter to Southeast Asia and Australia, part of them travel up the west coast towards the American continent (OLSEN et al., 2006).

Recently, a study based on the phylogenetic analysis of the H6 subtype of the AI virus (which frequently occurs in domestic and wild birds in Asia, North America and Africa) showed that the Eurasian subtype invaded North America several years ago, with the first introductions occurring 10 years before the first detections of these viruses.

isolates. The samples surveyed showed that the American strain, which accounted for 100% in 1980, decreased to 20% in 2000, being replaced by samples of Eurasian origin (DOHNA et al., 2009).

3.7 Bird migrations in North America

North America has several migratory routes traveled by a large number of birds. Stretching from the Arctic border, it covers extensive forest areas (Tundra and Boreal), alternates dry and wet areas, comprising a large breeding area for millions of migratory birds - some species that occur on other continents and others that are unique to the New World. This climatic diversity allows for the occurrence of long summer days with abundant food and long winter nights with extremely low temperatures and little food availability (ELPHICK, 2007).

The migratory routes of birds on the North American continent are numerous, with some being easy to trace and others extremely complicated. Some of the factors that make this diversity possible include the difference in the distance traveled, the start of the migration, the speed of flight, the geographical position and latitude of the breeding and wintering area, among others. Not only do two species from the same geographical area not follow the same migratory route from start to finish, but two groups of the same species from the same origin can also follow different migratory routes (BIRDNATURE, 2009). In addition, birds can move in an east-west direction or diagonally, finding another migratory route and moving south. Some migratory species or even the population of a particular species has a defined migration path, which can determine which migratory route is used. However, many species have a very broad movement pattern that does not fit into any defined migratory route pattern (ELPHICK, 2007).

The migration of North American birds normally takes place in a north-south direction, with a greater concentration on the ocean coasts, along mountain ranges and in the valleys of the main rivers. This means that a major migratory route is close to a particular topographical feature that does not prevent movement in a north-south direction (BIRDNATURE, 2009).

The main migratory routes on the North American continent are: the Atlantic, the Mississippi, the Central and the Pacific (Figures 33 and 34). With the exception of the routes along the ocean coasts, the main migratory routes overlap as they move north-south, with parts of all four of the main routes emerging as one towards the south around Panama (BIRDNATURE, 2009).

Approximately 80% of the species and 94% of the individuals that reproduce in northern coniferous forests migrate to the tropics. In the deciduous forests of northeastern America, 62% of the species and 75% of the individuals that breed in this environment also migrate. In the central plains, 76% of breeding species and 73% of individuals are migrants. Among the bird populations that breed in the west and south of the continent, the percentage of migrants declines considerably (ELPHICK, 2007).

Of the bird species that breed in the United States and Canada (around 650 species), approximately 130 (20%) are non-migratory. However, many of these birds make local seasonal movements, such as moving from high to low areas in the mountains or dispersing from breeding areas to other areas that are not breeding sites. Non-migratory bird species include many woodpeckers, grouse and some owls, whose occurrence is limited to warmer areas (ELPHICK, 2007).

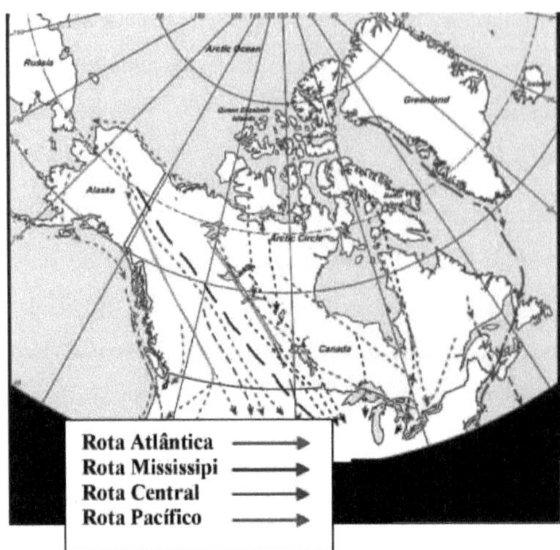

Figure 33 - Main migratory routes for birds in Canada.

Source: BIRDNATURE (2009).

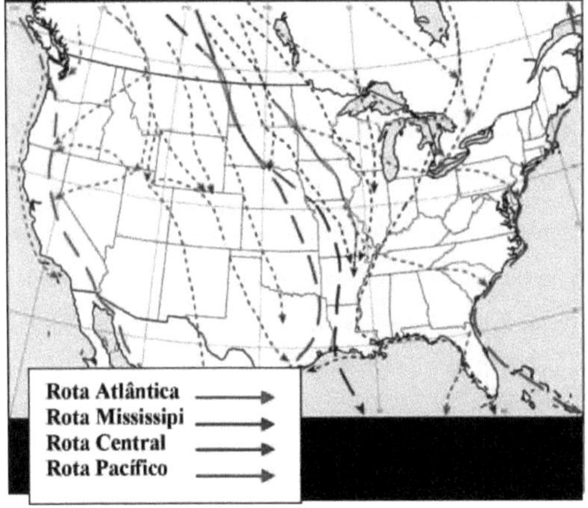

Figure 34 - Main migratory routes for birds in the USA.

Source: BIRDNATURE (2009).

For some birds, the Florida peninsula, passing through the Antilles, is the reference route for migrants from South America. For other species, Florida itself, the Bahamas and the Caribbean Islands serve as a refuge from the harsh winter. The northern coast of the Gulf of Mexico represents a mountainous barrier to southbound migrants, bifurcating their passage to the east or west. For others, it serves as a food and rest stop to continue their journey to their final destination (ELPHICK, 2007).

Two other migratory bird routes should be considered, involving other continents such as Europe,

Asia, Africa and Oceania (Figure 35). The first is the Asian-Australian route, which extends from the Arctic circle of Siberia and eastern Alaska, north and southeast Asia, to Australia and New Zealand. It covers twenty-two countries including Alaska (USA), Japan, Russia, China, Taiwan, North Korea, South Korea, Malaysia, Thailand, Vietnam, Philippines, Indonesia, Mongolia, Cambodia, Myanmar, Bangladesh, East Timor, Brunei, Singapore, Papua New Guinea, Australia and New Zealand. Approximately 55 species of birds use this migratory route, mainly from the Charadriiformes order (38 species). Included in this order are 28 species from the Scolopacidae family, eight from the Charadriidae family and two from the Scolopacidae family (BIRD FLU, 2009). It should be noted that among the species of the Charadriiform Order that use this migratory route, 10 species also occur in Brazil (CBRO, 2009).

The second is the Atlantic Route, which passes through Africa, enters western and eastern Europe, reaches northern Canada and arrives in the eastern portion of the Hudson River Bay, in the direction of the Canadian Maritime Provinces (BIRD FLU, 2009).

These two routes intersect the north-south routes from North America to South America. They can thus reach the central region of Canada, the United States and South America (BIRD FLU, 2009).

3.8 Bird migrations to Brazil from North America

In a study by Sick (1983) on migratory birds in South America, the author divided the movements that occur on this continent into: nearshore migrations (when the birds come from North America); southern migrations (northward movements of birds from the southern hemisphere); regional, local or partial movements (movements of limited distance, as a result of the seasonality of water and trophic resources); movements from the Andes and in the mountain ranges east of Brazil (producing important altitudinal migrations).

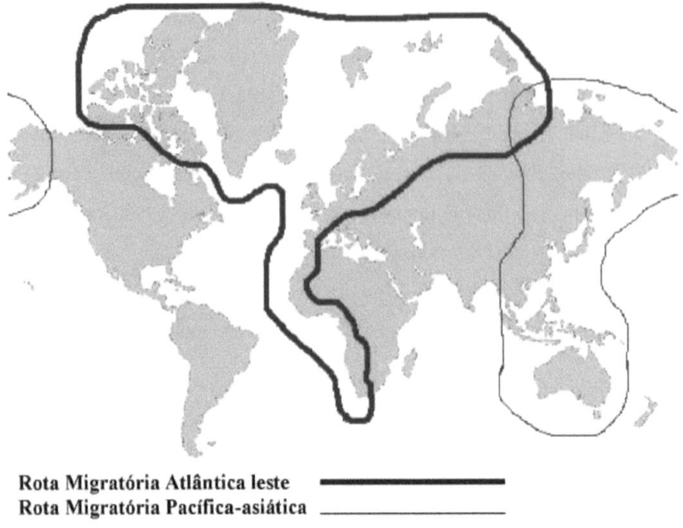

Figure 35 - Migration routes covering the American, African, Asian, European and Oceania continents.

Source: BIRD FLU (2009).

In the case of Neotropical migrants, more than 420 species migrate to the Neotropics, predominantly in Central America and decreasing towards the south. Among the migrant groups, the Passeriformes prefer Central America and the Caribbean, while the non-Passeriformes are more widely distributed (STOTZ et al., 1996 apud ALVES, 2007).

Nearshore migrants have wider geographic distributions and greater habitat tolerances than resident species, and can use secondary habitats such as pine forests and secondary forests and coastal habitats (STOTZ et al., 1996 apud ALVES, 2007).

In Brazil, the northern migrants enter through the northern part of the country (Figure 36). In fact, the Amazon and the coastal zone of the North and Northeast regions are places where there are many records of these visitors, generally arriving in the country between August and October and returning to their breeding areas between March and May (NUNES et al., 2006).

The Charadriiformes (curlews, batuiras, gulls and thirty-réis) correspond to the most representative group of birds among the nearshore migrants, which are characterized by gathering in large groups and making long continental journeys, originating from the most extreme portions of the American continent. Most of the movements take place along the country's coastline, with the most important ones in the North: the salt flats of Pará, the coast of Amapà and the reentrances of Maranhão; in the Northeast, the coast of the states of Rio Grande do Norte, Pernambuco, Sergipe and Bahia; and in the South, the Lagoa do Peixe National Park, in Rio Grande do Sul. However, part of the population, after passing through Venezuela and Colombia, reaches the Amazon through the eastern part, following the route of the great rivers (Rio Negro, Branco and Madeira) (SICK, 2003). Also in the west, they follow the Araguaia and Xingu rivers into central Brazil, continuing as far south as Tierra del Fuego (NUNES et al., 2006).

There is also another group of migrant birds from North America that arrive in Brazil, including teals, raptors, bacuraus, cuckoos, swallows and passerines (parulideos, embrezideos, tiranideos, turdideos, icterideos, and hirundinideos). Most of these species follow migratory routes within the continent that overlap when they pass through Central America or the Caribbean islands, reaching the coast of Colombia. Among the passerines, the swallows stand out because of their large groups (hundreds or thousands), which are found in large numbers in the Amazon.

The four migrant species that arrive in Brazil from September onwards are the blue swallow (*Progne subis*), the barranco swallow (*Riparia riparia*), the flock swallow (*Hirundo rustica*) and the ring-billed swallow (*Petrochelidon pyrronota*) (NUNES et al., 2006). These species of passerine birds, which breed in the high latitudes of the northern hemisphere, migrate in a southerly direction, passing through the Amazon and making their way to the south and southeast of Brazil, and may even reach Argentina (NUNES et al., 2006).

In general, studies of passerine migrations on the American continent, including Brazil, are poorly understood. There is also the fact that some species migrate at night, have their plumage sexually resting and do not emit sound signals during the wintering period, making it difficult to identify them (NUNES et al., 2006). In most cases, the main reason for animal species seeking Brazil during the winter is not the higher temperatures of the tropics and subtropics; what brings them to the country is the greater availability of food due to the warm and rainy climate (SICK, 1983).

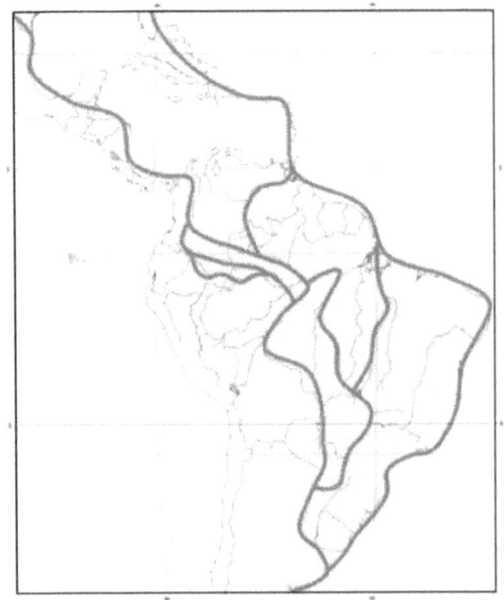

Figure 36 - Main migratory routes for birds arriving in Brazil from North America.

Source: NUNES et al. (2006).

4 SANITARY DEFENSE SYSTEM FOR THE PREVENTION AND CONTROL OF AVIAN INFLUENZA

4.1 National Poultry Health Program

Current legislation supports measures to prevent, control and eradicate exotic and emergency diseases (including Avian Influenza). This legislative framework includes Ministerial Ordinance No. 193, of September 19, 1994, which institutes the National Poultry Health Program (PNSA) and creates its advisory committee; Normative Instruction of the Agricultural Defense System (SDA) No. 32, of May 13, 2002, which approves the Technical Surveillance Standards for Newcastle disease and avian influenza; SDA Normative Instruction No. 17, of April 7, 2006, which approves the National Plan for the Prevention of Avian Influenza and the Control and Prevention of Newcastle disease throughout the national territory. The Animal Health Defense Service (SDSA), which is run by the Animal Defense Secretariat of the Ministry of Agriculture, Livestock and Food Supply (MAPA), through Article 63 of the SDSA Regulations (Decree No. 24.548 of July 3, 1934) and Law No. 569 of December 21, 1948, establish the measures to be applied in the event of Avian Influenza being found in poultry flocks, including the sacrifice of birds and compensation for owners, where appropriate (BRASIL, 2009); Ministerial Normative Instruction No. 56, of December 4, 2007, establishes the procedures for registering, inspecting and controlling breeding and commercial poultry establishments Normative Instruction 56 was recently replaced by Normative Instruction 59, of December 2, 2009.

Normative Instruction No. 32 of the SDA defines, among several actions listed, the obligatory notification to the official veterinary service of the occurrence of symptoms suggestive of Newcastle Disease and Avian Influenza in any species of bird; the carrying out of an immediate investigation at the suspect establishment by the official veterinary doctor; the collection of material from suspect birds and their forwarding to the official laboratory; restricting the movement of birds and their products from suspect establishments; establishing a protection zone (a radius of 3 km) and a surveillance zone (a radius of 10 km) (Figure 37) around the suspect establishment; controlling the movement of people in risk areas; sacrificing all infected birds; cleaning and disinfecting facilities and vehicles; and properly disposing of carcasses and other waste (Figure 38) (BRASIL, 2002).

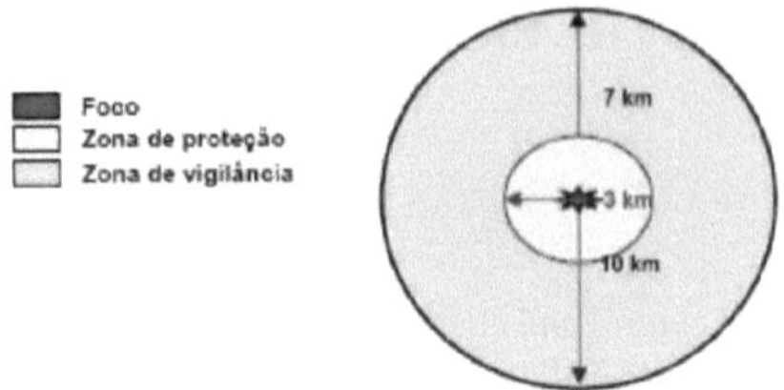

Figure 37 - Division of the affected area into protection and surveillance zones from the focus. Source: BRASIL (2002).

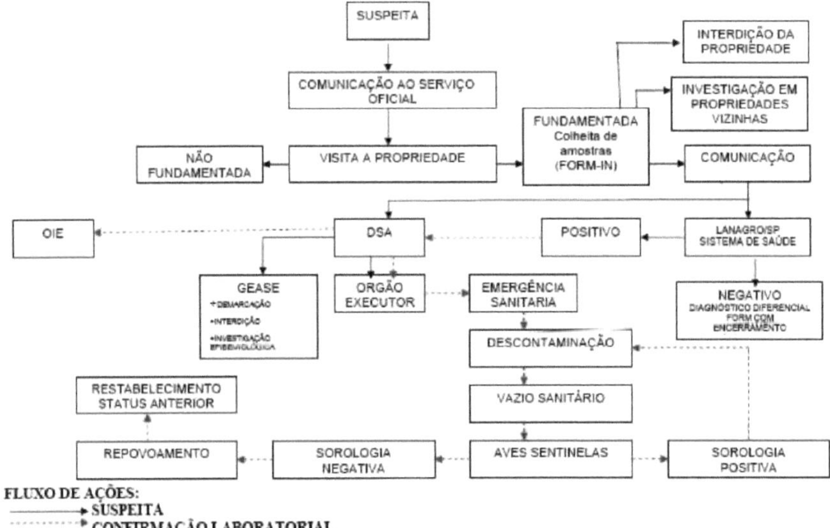

Figure 38 - Flowchart of actions in the event of suspected Avian Influenza.

Source: BRASIL (2002).

Subsequently, Normative Instruction 17 of the SDA approved the National Plan for the Prevention of Avian Influenza and Newcastle Disease, as part of the PNSA, defining the responsibilities of the public and private bodies involved in the plan. Brazilian states join the Plan on a voluntary basis and the criteria contained in this normative instruction are used to evaluate and classify the health services of the federation units. Among the criteria assessed for the classification are descriptive data on the state's poultry industry, the veterinary care system, conditions for responding to health emergencies and compliance with the PNSA standards, through audits carried out by MAPA (BRASIL, 2009a). As a result, four groups are defined which, in order of best classification, receive a grade from A to D. The audits and respective classifications were carried out in 2007 and 2008. The main weaknesses found in the 2008 audits were: deficiencies in passive and active surveillance, low notification of suspected poultry diseases, failures to respond to notified suspicions, a lack of human and material resources in the PNSA area, a lack of specific training and a lack of state financial resources for poultry health activities. In the 2007 and 2008 audits, no Brazilian state obtained an A rating for its health services (Figure 39). Only Paranà, Santa Catarina and Mato Grosso received a B rating in the 2008 audit. This year, Minas Gerais received a C rating in the audit carried out, with improvements needed mainly in the veterinary care system and in the ability to respond to health emergencies (BRASIL, 2006).

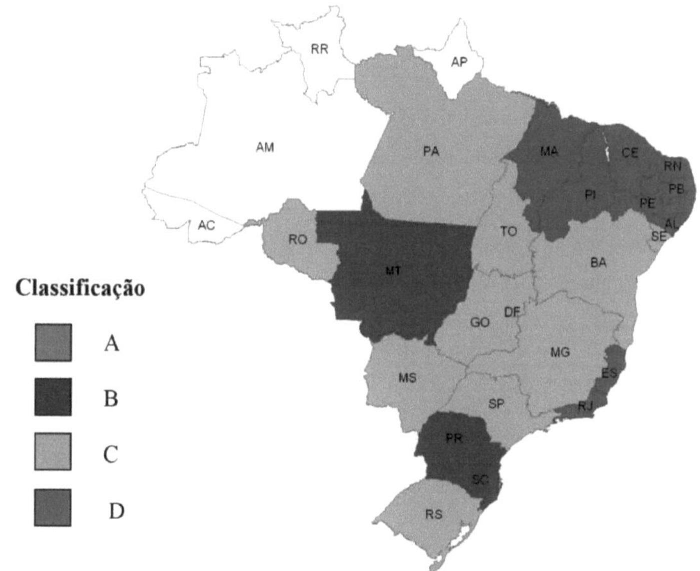

Figure 39 - Results of the PNSA assessments in the 2008 audits.

Source: BRASIL (2009a).

With the aim of improving the evaluation of its health services system in the poultry sector in the state of Minas Gerais, the Group for Special Veterinary Care in Poultry (GAVEA) was created. Made up of 14 veterinarians from the Instituto Mineiro de Agropecuària (IMA), the state's official animal and plant health agency, they will work exclusively with poultry in the regional coordinating offices where there is a high concentration of poultry, namely: Bambui, Juiz de Fora, Oliveira, Passos, Patrocinio, Uberaba, Uberlândia, Varginha and Viçosa. Re-registering poultry farms, dealing with suspected notifiable diseases, registering establishments that sell live poultry and registering other poultry farms are some of the activities that the Group intends to carry out (IMA, 2009).

Ministerial Normative Instruction No. 59, which recently replaced MAPA Normative Instruction No.

56, defines a series of biosecurity measures to be observed and inspected in industrial poultry farms (BRASIL, 2009b).

As part of these measures, Article 10 establishes minimum distances between the location of poultry establishments and other places that pose risks to the health and well-being of birds or to the quality of their products (BRASIL, 2009b).

Articles 11, 12, 13 and 14 stipulate that poultry houses must be protected from the outside environment by installing screens with a mesh size of less than 2 cm, to prevent birds, domestic animals and wild animals from entering (Figure 40). It also stipulates that the floor must be made of masonry and that the building must allow the internal surfaces to be washed and disinfected (BRASIL, 2009b).

Another requirement of this normative instruction is that, according to articles 15, 16, 17 and 18, poultry establishments must have specific facilities, such as changing rooms, toilets and others, according to the type of poultry farm (BRASIL, 2009b).

The entry of people unrelated to the production process into poultry establishments must also be monitored. According to Article 20, some prior procedures must be adopted, such as bathing and changing clothes and shoes (BRASIL, 2009b).

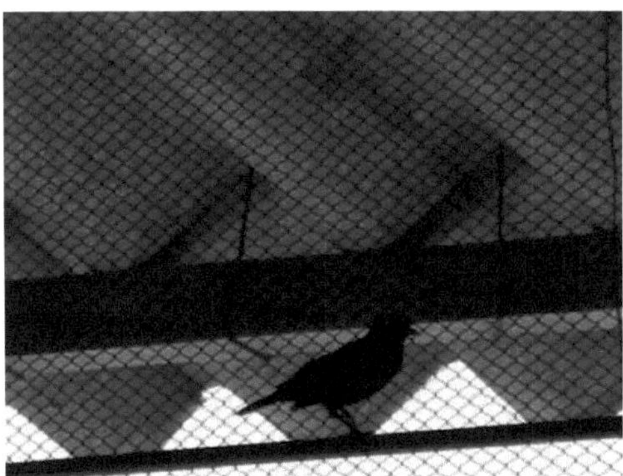

Figure 40 - Use of bird screens and devices to prevent birds from entering the poultry house.

Source: REZENDE (2007).

Water and animal feed must be treated in such a way as to eliminate the possibility of introducing pathogens to the animals, as explained in Article 19 (Figure 41).

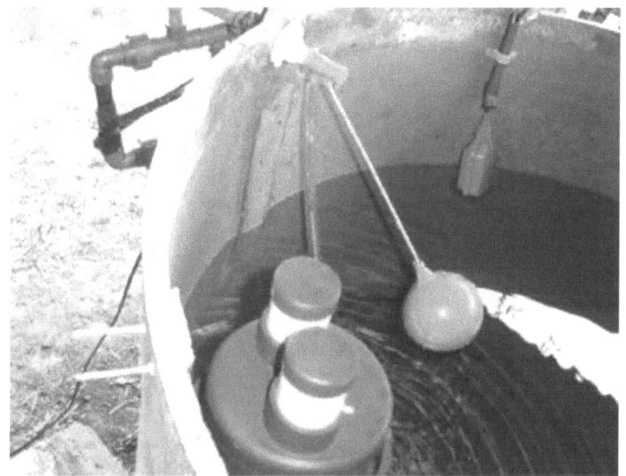

Figure 41 - Water treatment in the water tank with chlorine.

Source: REZENDE (2007).

Other important measures were also included, such as controlling the transit of people and vehicles (Art. 21, I), protecting establishments with security fences (Art. 21, II), disinfecting vehicles at the entrance and exit of poultry establishments (Art. 21, III) (Figure 42), washing and disinfecting facilities between each poultry rearing cycle (Art. 21, VI), monitoring various diseases, including those with a public health impact, such as AI (Art. 22, 23 and 23), and adopting a vaccination program. 21, VI), the monitoring of various diseases, including those with an impact on public health, such as AI (arts. 22, 23 and 24) and the adoption of a vaccination program in accordance with the specific health challenges of each region and with the use of products duly registered with MAPA (BRASIL, 2009b).

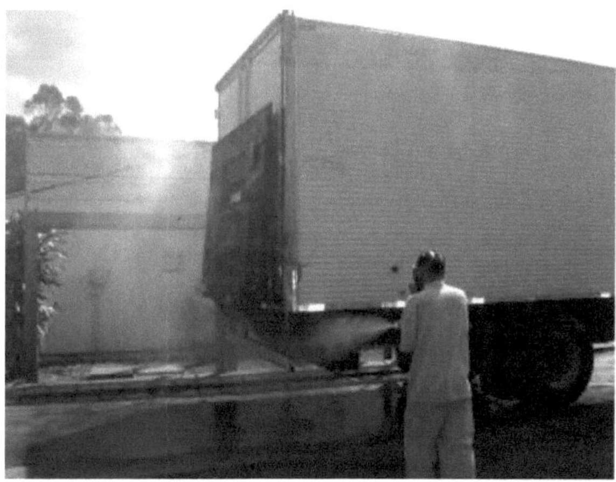

Figure 42 - Washing and disinfecting vehicles entering farms.

Source: REZENDE (2007).

4.2 Simulated Exercise on the Introduction of a Highly Pathogenic Virus in the State of Minas Gerais

The simulated AI introduction exercise held in Uberaba, Minas Gerais, provided participants with better preparation and knowledge of the emergency measures that must be taken to control and eradicate the disease. At the end of the meeting, the potential risks of the introduction of the IAAP virus in the Triângulo Mineiro region of Minas Gerais were raised:

- Goods and products that can be vehicles for the risk of the IAAP virus entering the countryside: the import of contaminated hatching eggs, the transit of commercial eggs and live birds (breeders, broilers, turkeys, ostriches, free-range birds), the interstate transit of birds for slaughter, the transportation of ornamental birds, the transit of by-products (poultry litter), migratory bird routes, the breeding of carrier pigeons, clandestine slaughterhouses, wild birds and cockfighting.

- People who may be the primary risk generators or agents: international visitors (from risk areas), veterinarians, extension workers, tax agents, truck drivers, suppliers of goods and inputs and hunting and fishing activities.

- The main entry points for the virus: airports, highways, railroads, zoos, ponds and reservoirs.

- Consequences with an economic impact following the introduction of the IAAP virus: the suspension of exports, the sacrifice of a large number of birds, the loss of profitability for the industry, the volume of poultry meat on offer far exceeding demand (restriction of consumption and drop in poultry housing), the inflation of other protein sources (beef, pork, for example), the indebtedness of rural producers, among others.

- Assessment of the current development of prevention activities and the infrastructure of the official surveillance system: lacking in terms of staff and material resources.

- Possible "niches" of infection in the state: zoos, dams and ponds, urban birds (pigeons, sparrows) and pigsties.

4.3 Training Private Sector Technicians

The private sector is an integral part of the National Plan for the Prevention of Avian Influenza and the Control and Prevention of Newcastle Disease, in accordance with SDA Normative Instruction No. 56 (art. 5, item VI). Paragraph 8 of Article 5 of the plan establishes that:

"... I - immediately report any suspected presence of Avian Influenza and Newcastle Disease to the Official Service and carry out the necessary actions to fully investigate the case;

II - encourage the development of private state funds, recognized by MAPA, to carry out emergency actions in the event of an outbreak of Avian Influenza and Newcastle Disease, in commercial poultry farms or not, including the possibility of paying compensation;

III - promote continuing education programs for veterinarians, technicians and poultry producers, in accordance with the PNSA manuals; (emphasis added)

IV - participate in the State Poultry Health Committee and in the actions of the State Poultry Health Emergency Groups;

V - adopt minimum biosecurity actions, defined by the PNSA, in commercial poultry establishments." (BRAZIL, 2007).

In this sense, the technicians of the country's main poultry companies have taken part in training courses on emergency diseases, whether promoted by official bodies or those organized internally (Figures 43 and 44).

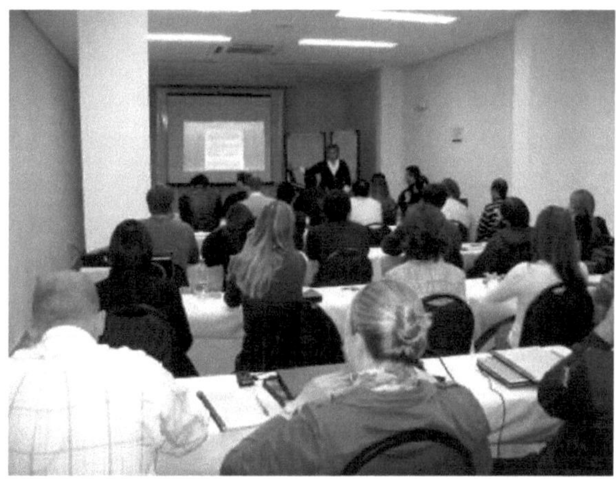

Figure 43 - Theoretical training course on emergency illnesses held in a private company. Source: REZENDE (2007).

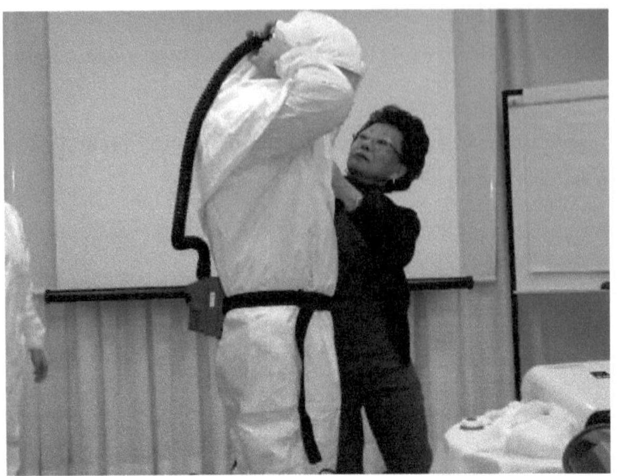

Figure 44 - Practical training in emergency illnesses at a private company. Source: REZENDE (2007).

4.4 Health System of the Municipality of Uberlândia

The definition of indices such as the number of beds or doctors per inhabitant depends on regional, socio-economic, cultural and epidemiological factors, among others, which are different between countries or even between regions of the same country. However, there is a better ratio of doctors to inhabitants in some countries (mainly in the Scandinavian countries, Spain, Argentina and Uruguay) (Table 17). With regard to the number of beds per inhabitant, Japan has the best ratio, while Finland, Argentina, the United Kingdom and Denmark also have superior results. It is worth noting that countries which have had human cases of Avian Influenza (Thailand, Vietnam), in addition to having a low number of doctors per inhabitant, have also shown, in comparison with the others, a low number of beds per inhabitant (Table 17) (WHO, 2009).

Table 17

Number of doctors and hospital beds per 1,000 inhabitants (WHO, 2009).

Parents	Number of Doctors	Number of beds
Argentina	3,0	4,1
Bolivia	1,2	1,1
Brazil	1,2	2,4
Canada	1,9	3,4
Chile	1,1	2,3
China	1,4	2,2
Denmark	3,6	3,8
Spain	3,3	3,4
United States	2,6	3,1
Finland	3,3	6,8
Japan	2,1	14,0
United Kingdom	2,3	3,9
Thailand	0,4	2,2
Vietnam	0,6	2,7

Uruguay	3,7	2,9

Source: WHO (2009).

The city of Uberlândia has 912 establishments registered in the National Register of Health Establishments (CNES), including general and specialized hospitals, health posts, isolated practices, specialized clinics and other establishments of the same kind. The hospital network has one public hospital for medium and high complexity care and four private hospitals, one of which provides medium and high complexity care and the others medium complexity. (UBERLÂNDIA, 2008).

With an estimated population of just over 630,000 inhabitants, the CNES registered 2,133 doctors working in the city in 2007, and health establishments offered 1,226 beds, 766 of which were in the SUS network (BRASIL, 2008).

5 FINAL CONSIDERATIONS

To date, *there* have been no reports of highly pathogenic avian influenza in Brazil. Despite the periodic flow of migratory birds, epidemiological investigations carried out in some migratory sites have indicated the presence of low pathogenic avian influenza. The country is therefore considered to be at low risk of IAAP.

Brazil has a good health defense program for the prevention and eradication of emergency diseases. There is still a need for greater progress in adapting the number of people in the official service, providing it with greater material resources. Private companies in the poultry sector play an important role in the National Poultry Health Program as participants in its implementation.

The rural survey of the municipality of Uberlândia, Minas Gerais, showed that 44.42% of rural properties in the municipality of Uberlândia raise poultry, 73% of which are subsistence poultry, known as caipiras, corresponding to 0.62% of the municipality's poultry population.

Subsistence farming is carried out without the adoption of basic health safety criteria, mostly in an open environment, and the birds are subject to the possibility of infection by pathogens from wild birds living in the same place. A possible contamination of these birds with the avian influenza virus would result in the transmission of this agent to subsistence poultry. These birds would represent a threat of transmission of the IAAP virus to industrial poultry.

There is a proximity between farms that raise free-range poultry and farms that raise industrial poultry. Although legislation sets minimum distance criteria for industrial breeding facilities, the same requirements are not applied to free-range poultry.

The survey of the avifauna around the Amador Aguiar I and II hydroelectric dams identified the occurrence of migratory bird species from North America, a region with a history of avian influenza virus occurrences. Although there are migratory birds around the hydroelectric plants, it is not known whether they have had contact with the AI virus.

A possible occurrence of avian influenza in any region of Brazil would collapse the entire chicken meat production chain, with repercussions from grain production to industrial activity, including a halt to exports and a sharp drop in domestic consumption of chicken meat. As this is a disease with a public health impact, it would also represent the risk of an epidemic, exposing a large number of poultry workers to the risk of infection.

Considering the criteria for choosing migratory sites for active AI surveillance, areas with water reservoirs (such as hydroelectric dams) and with the presence of migratory bird species should be included in the AI epidemiological investigation program. Especially when the birds come from places at risk of the disease and the areas receiving the migratory birds have a significant domestic population, as well as wild birds.

The area surrounding the Amador Aguiar I and II hydroelectric dams should also be considered a low-risk region for the introduction of avian influenza. Considering the presence of migratory birds from North America, living in the same environment as wild birds and free-range birds, which in turn are close to the poultry farms of industrial establishments, there is a need to carry out an epidemiological survey of migratory birds.

The public animal health service, run at federal level by the Ministry of Agriculture, Livestock and Supply, needs to regulate the conditions under which subsistence poultry is reared in the country, implementing measures that are compatible with maintaining the health status of industrial poultry, also having repercussions on the prevention of zoonoses, with an impact on public health.

6 REFERENCES

ABEF. Brazilian Association of Chicken Exporters. **Annual Report 2008/2009.** Available at: <http://www.abef.com.br/portal>. Accessed on October 13, 2009.

ALVES, M. A. S. Bird migration systems in terrestrial environments in Brazil: examples, gaps and proposals for advancing knowledge. **Revista Brasileira de Ornitologia.** Sao Paulo, v. 15, n. 2, jun.2007, p. 231-238. Available at: <http://www.ecoaves.uerj.br/documents/Alves_RevBrasOrnit2007.pdf>. Accessed on: 22.mar.2009.

ASSUNÇÂO, W. L.; LIMA, S. do C.; ROSA, R. Preliminary approach to the climatic conditions of Uberlândia (MG). **Revista Sociedade e Natureza,** Uberlândia, v. 3, n. 5 e 6, p. 91 - 107, jan.- dez. 1991.

AVIBASE. **The world bird database.** Available at: < http://avibase.bsc- eoc.org/species.jsp>. Accessed on: 22.nov.2008

AZEVEDO JÛNIOR, Severino Mendes. Migratory birds and avian influenza in Brazil. In: **Revista do Conselho Federal de Medicina Veterinària**, Brasilia, v. 12, n. 37 p. 80, jan.-abr. 2006.

BACCARO, C. A. D.; MEDEIROS, S. M. de; FERREIRA, I. L.; RODRIGUES, S. C. Geomorphological mapping of the Araguari River Basin (MG). In: LIMA, S. do C.;

SANTOS, R. J. (Org.). **Environmental management of the Araguari River Basin - Towards sustainable development.** Uberlândia: EDUFU, 2003. p. 1-19.

BECKER, B.; UYS, C.J. Experimental infection of chickens with influenza A/Tern/South Africa/1961 and Chicken/Scotland/1959 viruses : II. Pathology. **Journal of Comparative Pathology.** South Africa, v. 77, n. 2, apr.1967, 167-172 p. Available at: <http://www.sciencedirect.com/science?_ob=ArticleURL&_udi=B6WHW-4DCW0WB-4F&_user=10&_rdoc=1&_fmt=&_orig=search&_sort=d&_docanchor=&view=c&_searchStrId=1124509861&_rerunOrigin=google&_acct=C000050221&_version=1&_urlVersion=0&_userid=10&md5=3db9ca416b8b56e716ff354ab46a4b25>. Accessed on October 26, 2009.

BIRD NATURE. **North American Migration Flyways.** Available at: <http://www.birdnature.com/flyways.html>. Accessed on: 22.Apr.2009.

BIRD FLU. **Bird Migration Paths.** Available at: <http//www.birdfluclues/flyways.html.> .comAccessed on: 07.May.2009.

BOREAL BIRDS. BOREAL SONGBIRD INITIATIVE. **Birds of the Boreal Forest.**

Available at: <

http://www.borealbirds.org/guide/guide_detail.php?curr_rec=118&view=imagelist&guideid=1&groupid=1&familyid=&term=&process=1&sort=&from=108>. Accessed on: 01.nov.2008.

BORGES, M.R.; RODRIGUES, P.O.; MELO, C. Avifauna associated with four ponds in the city of Uberlândia, MG. In: **XVI BRAZILIAN CONGRESS OF ORNITHOLOGY,** 2008. Abstracts ...Palmas: Universidade Federal de Tocantis, 2008. p. 186.

BRAZIL. Ministry of Agriculture, Livestock and Supply. **National Poultry Health Program - PNSA.** Available at: <http://www.agricultura.gov.br/>. Accessed on: 08.oct.2009.

. **Normative Instruction No. 32, of May 13, 2002.** Available at: <http://www.agricultura.gov.br/.> Accessed on: 06.nov.2009.

. **Normative Instruction No. 17, of April 7, 2007.** Available at: <http://www.agricultura.gov.br/.> Accessed on: 06.nov.2009.

.. **Sanitary Surveillance: National Poultry Health Program.** Available at: <http://www.uba.org.br/site3/sanidade_avicola/pnsa_rt_jul_2009_regina_d_arce.pdf.> Accessed on: October 26, 2009a.

. **Normative Instruction No. 59, of December 2, 2009.** Available at: <http://www.agricultura.gov.br/.> Accessed on: 06.Dec.2009b.

BRAZIL. Ministry of Health. **Revista Saùde, Brasil**. Brasilia, v.3, n.1, December 2006.

Available at: <http: //portal.saude.gov.br/portal/arquivos/pdf/saudebrasil_dezembro2006.pdf.> Accessed on: 04.Apr.2009.

. **Epidemiological Electronic Bulletin.** Brasilia, n. 2, 19.02.2004, 2 p. Available at: http://portal.saude.gov.br/portal/arquivos/pdf/Boletim_eletronico_02_ano04.pdf.

Accessed on: 16.nov.2008.

. **National Register of Health Establishments (CNES).** Available at: <http://cnes.datasus.gov.br/Mod_Ind_Tipo_Leito.asp>. Accessed on: 30.nov.2009

CAPUA, I.; ALEXANDER, D. J. Ecology, Epidemiology and Human Health implications of Avian Influenza Virus Infections. **Avian Influenza and Newcastle Disease.** Milan: Springer, 2009. p. 1-18.

CBRO. BRAZILIAN COMMITTEE OF ORNITHOLOGICAL RECORDS. **Lists of the birds of Brazil.** Version 05/10/2008. Available at <http://www.cbro.org.br>. Accessed on: 01.feb.2009.

CDC. United States of America Center for Disease Control and Prevention. **CDC**

Estimates of 2009 H1N1 Influenza Cases, Hospitalizations and Deaths in the United States, April - October 17, 2009 Available at: <http://www.cdc.gov/h1n1flu/estimates_2009_h1n1.htm> Accessed on: 06.nov.2009.

CAPIM BRANCO ENERGY CONSORTIUM. **General information about CCBE.** Available at: <http://www.ccbe.com.br/home/?page_id=2>. Accessed on: 02.05.2009.

CORNELL LAB OF ORNITHOLOGY. **All about Birds.** Available at: < http://www.allaboutbirds.org/guide>. Accessed on: 01.nov.2008.

COTTA, T. **Broiler chickens: breeding, slaughtering and marketing.** Viçosa: Aprenda Fàcil, 2003. 237 p.

DOHNA, H; LI, J.; CARDONA, C.J.; MILER, J.; CARPENTER, T.E. Invasions by Eurasian Avian Influenza Virus H6 Genes and Replacement of Its North American Clade.

Emergent Infect Diseases, v. 15, n. 7, july 2009, p. 1040-1045. Available at: <http://www.ncbi.nlm.nih.gov/pmc/articles/PMC2744232/pdf/09-0245_finalR.pdf.> Accessed on September 21, 2009.

ELPHICK, J. **Atlas of Bird Migration: tracing the great journeys of the world's birds.**

Buffalo: Firefly books, 2007, 176 p.

FAO. FOOD AND AGRICULTURE ORGANIZATION OF THE UNITED NATIONS. **Preparing for Highly Pathogenic Avian Influenza.** New York, n. 3, rev. ed., 94 p. Available at: <ftp://ftp.fao.org/docrep/fao/012/i0808e/i0808e.pdf> Accessed on: 26.nov.2009.

FAUCI, Anthony S.; MORENS, David M.; TAUBENBERGER, Jeffery K. The Persistent Legacy of the 1918 Influenza Virus. In: **The New England Journal of Medicine,** Whaltan-MA, v. 361, n. 3, p. 225-229, july 2009. Available at: < http://content.nejm.org/cgi/content/short/361/3/225>. Accessed on: 09.oct.2009.

HALVORSON, D.A. Prevention and Management of Avian Influenza outbreaks: experiences from the United States of America. **Review Scientific and Technical of the Office International Epizootie.** Paris, v. 28, n. 1, 2009, p. 359-369. Available at: < http://www.oie.int/boutique/extrait/halvorson359370.pdf>. Accessed on: October 11, 2009.

IMA. Minas Gerais Institute of Agriculture. **What happens at the IMA.** Available at: <http://www.ima.mg.gov.br/acontece-no-ima/558-grupo-de-trabalho-reforca-sanidade- avicola-em-minas.> Accessed on: 26.Sep.2009.

JONES, Kate E.; PATEL, Nikkita G.; LEVY, Marc A.; STOEYGARD, Adam; BALK, Deborah;

GITTLEMAN, John L. ; DASZAK, Peter. Global trends in emerging infectious diseases. In: **NATURE,** New York, v. 451, n. 21, p. 990-993, feb. 2008. Available at: <http://www.nature.com/nature/journal/v451/n7181/abs/nature06536.html>. Accessed on: October 12, 2009.

KHALAKDINA, A.; NARAIN, J. P. Avian Influenza: Responding to the Pandemic Threat. WHO. WORLD HEALTH ORGANIZATION. **Regional Health Forum,** v.9, n. 2, 2005. Available at:

<http://www.searo.who.int/LinkFiles/Regional_Health_Forum_Volume_9_No_2_avianinfl uenza.pdf>. Accessed on: 05.02.2009.

KISHIBE, R.; CANCHERINI, L. C. GOULART, V. S.; BERTECHINI, A. G.;

FASSANI, E.J. **Manual da Produçâo de Aves caipiras.** Lavras: Available at: <http://www.editora.ufla.br/BolExtensao/pdfBE/bol_05.pdf. Accessed on: 10.06.2009

KRAUSS, S.; WALKER, D.; PRYOR, S. P.; NILES, L.; CHENGHONG, L.; HINSHAW, V.S.; WEBSTER, R.G. Influenza A viruses in migrating wild aquatic birds in North America. **Vector-Borne and Zoonotic Diseases,** v. 4, n.3, 2004, p. 177-189. Available at: <http://www.ncbi.nlm.nih.gov/pubmed/15631061>. Accessed on: 08.08.2009.

MANNA & TOLEDO ENVIRONMENTAL PLANNING LTDA. **Final Report**

-Project to Confirm the Presence of Threatened Species at the Amador Aguiar I and II Hydroelectric Power Plants" - Monitoring Program for Endangered Winged and Terrestrial Fauna Phase I (Species Confirmation). Uberlândia: March, 2008. 178p.

MENDES, A. A.; SALDANHA, E. S. P. B. The poultry meat production chain in Brazil. In: MENDES, A. A.; NAAS, I. A.; MACARI, M (Org.). **Broiler Production.** Campinas: FACTA, 2004. p. 1 - 22.

MILLER, MARK A.; VIBOUD, Cecile; BALINSKA, Marta; SIMONSEN, Lone. The Signature Features of Influenza Pandemics - Implications for Policy. In: **The New England Journal of Medicine,** Whaltan-MA, v. 360, n. 25. p. 2595-2598, june 2009. Available at: < http://content.nejm.org/cgi/content/short/360/25/2595>. Accessed on: 09.oct.2009.

NUNES, M.F.C; LACERDA, R.; ROOS, A.; COSTA, J. **Migratory Birds in the Amazon and Avian Influenza.** CEMAVE. Information 35/2006 CEMAVE. Available at: <http://www.fmt.am.gov.br/imprensa/aves%20migratorias%20amazonia%20e%20gripe%2 0aviaria.pdf.> Accessed on July 6, 2007.

OIE. WORLD ANIMAL HEALTH ORGANIZATION. **Update on highly paghogenic avian influenza in animals (type H5 and H7).** Available at:

<http://www.oie.int/downld/AVIAN%20INFLUENZA/.htm>. Accessed on: 28.nov.2009a.

.. WORLD ANIMAL HEALTH ORGANIZATION. **Detailed country (ies) disease incidence.** Available at: < http://www.oie.int/wahis/public.php>. Accessed on: 24.nov.2009b.

OLSEN, B.; MUNSTER, V. J.; WALLENSTEN, A.; WALDENSTROM, J.; OSTERHAUS, A. D. M. E.; FOUCHIER, R. A. M. **Global patterns of influenza A virus in wild birds. Science,** v. 312, n. 5772, 21.apr.2006, p. 384-388. Available at: < http://www.sciencemag.org/cgi/content/full/312/5772/384.> Accessed on: 06.Dec.2008.

PASICK, J.; BERHANE, Y.; MCGREVY, K. H. Avian Influenza: the canadian experience. **Scientific and Technical Review of the Office International Epizootie.** Paris, v. 28, n. 1, 2009, p. 349-358. Available at: < http://www.oie.int/boutique/extrait/pasick349358.pdf>. Accessed on: October 11, 2009.

PEREIRA, M. S.; SILVA, P. L.. Prevalence of antibodies against Mycoplasma gallisepticum and Mycoplasma synoviae in free-range chickens in the municipality of Uberlândia - MG. **Revista Brasileira de Ciência Avicola / Brazilian Journal of Poultry Science,** Campinas, v. 7, n. Suplemento, p. 204-204, 2005a.

. Prevalence of antibodies against Salmonella Pullorum and bacteriological identification of Salmonella sp in free-range chickens in Uberlândia - MG. **Revista Brasileira de Ciência Avicola / Brazilian Journal of Poultry Science,** Campinas, v. 7, n. Suplemento, p. 205-205, 2005b.

REZENDE, M.S.; SILVA, P. L.; LIMA, S.C. Survey of the distances between industrial chicken and broiler farms and free-range poultry farms in the rural area of the municipality of Uberlândia, Minas Gerais. In: **FACTA Conference on Poultry Science and Technology 2008,** Santos: Agros, 2008. v. 10. p. 240-240.

ROWAN, W. Experiments in bird migration II. **Reversed migration.** Proc. Nat. Acad. Sci. v. 16, 1930, p. 520-525. apud ALVES, M. A. S. Bird migration systems in terrestrial environments in Brazil: examples, gaps and proposals for advancing knowledge. **Revista Brasileira de Ornitologia.** Sao Paulo, v. 15, n. 2, jun.2007, p. 231238. Available at: <http://www.ecoaves.uerj.br/documents/Alves_RevBrasOrnit2007.pdf>. Accessed on: 22.mar.2009.

SANO, S.M.; ALMEIDA, S.P. **Cerrado: environment and flora.** Planaltina: EMBRAPA- CDAC, 1998, 556 p.

SICK, H. **Migrations of birds in continental South America**. Brasilia: IBDF, 1983, 86p.

SILVA, E. M.; ASSUNÇÂO, W. L. . The climate in the city of Uberlândia - MG. **Revista Sociedade e Natureza,** Uberlândia, v. 30, p. 1-20, 2004.

STALLKNECHT, D. E. 1998. Ecology and epidemiology of avian influenza viruses in wild bird populations: Waterfowl, shorebirds, pelicans, cormorants, etc. SWAYNE, D.E. (Ed). In: **Proceedings of the fourth international symposium on avian influenza**, Kennett Square, American Association of Avian Pathologists, 1998, p. 61-69. Available at: <http://www.jstor.org/pss/3298801.> Accessed on: 03.07.2009

STALLKNECHT, D.E.; SHANE, S. M. 1988. Host range of avian influenza virus in free- living birds. **Veterinary Research Communications** 12: 125-141.

STALLKNECHT, D. E.; ZWANK, P.J.; SENNE, D.A.; KEARNEY. M.T. Avian influenza viruses from migratory and resident ducks of coastal Louisiana. **Avian Diseases.** v. 47, n.

3, 1990, p. 1107-1110. Available at:

<http://avdi.allenpress.com/avdionline/?request=get-abstract&doi=10.1637/0005-2086-47.s3.1107>. Accessed on 03.Jun.2009

STOTZ, D.F.; FITZPATRICK, J.W.; PARKER, T.A.; MOSKOVITZ, D.K. **Neotropical Birds: ecology and conservation.** The University of Chicago Press. USA. apud ALVES, M. A. S. Bird migration systems in terrestrial environments in Brazil: examples, gaps and proposals for advancing knowledge. **Revista Brasileira de Ornitologia.** Sao Paulo, v. 15, n. 2, jun.2007, p. 231-238. Available at: <http://www.ecoaves.uerj.br/documents/Alves_RevBrasOrnit2007.pdf>. Accessed on: 22.mar.2009.

TOLLIS, M; DI TRANI, L. Recent Developments in Avian Influenza Research: Epidemiology and Immunoprophylaxis. **The Veterinary Journal**. Maryland Heights, v. 164, p.202-215. 2002.

UBERLÂNDIA. City Hall. Municipal Department of Urban Planning and the Environment. **Integrated Database 2008.** v. 1. Available at: <http://www3.uberlandia.mg.gov.br/midia/documentos/planejamento_urbano/bdi_2008_vo l2.pdf>. Accessed on: 22.nov.2009.

VRANJAC, A. **Avian Influenza and Human Cases**. Revista Saùde Pùblica. Sao Paulo, v. 40, n.1, p.187-190, 2006.

WEBSTER, R.G; BEAN,W.J.; GORMAN, 0.T.; CHAMBERS, T.M.; KAWAOKA, Y. Evolution and Ecology of Influenza A Viruses. **Microbiological Review,** Washington, v. 56, n.1, p. 152-179, mar. 1992.

WHO. World Health Organization. **H5N1 avian influenza: timeline of major events.** Available at: <http://www.who.int/csr/disease/avian_influenza/ai_timeline/en/index>. Accessed on 01.Dec.2009.

Avian influenza: food safe issues. Available at:

<http://www.who.int/foodsafety/micro/avian/en/index.html>. Accessed on 01.Dec.2009.

. **Avian Influenza, Including Influenza A (H5N1) in Humans: WHO Interim Infection Control Guideline for Health Care Facilities.** Available at: < http://www.wpro.who.int/internet/resources.ashx/CSR/Publications/AI_Inf_Control_Guide_10May2007.pdf>. Accessed on: 08.03.2009

. **Cumulative Number of Confirmed Human Cases of Avian Influenza A/(H5N1) Reported to WHO.** Available at: <http://www.who.int/csr/disease/avian_influenza/country/cases_table_2009_11_27/en/index.html>. Accessed on: 08.Dec.2009.

. **Statistical Information System (WHOSIS).** Available at: <http://www.who.int/whosis/en/index.html>. Accessed on: 26.nov.2009.

. **Pandemic (H1N1) 2009 - Update 78** Available at: <http://www.who.int/csr/don/2009_12_11a/en/index.html>. Accessed on: 11.Dec.2009.

WORLD POULTRY. USAID **Program to Fight Zoonoses.** Available at: <http://www. worldpoultry.net>. Accessed on November 11, 2009.

ZANZARINI, R. M.; COSTA, R. S. Analysis of the impacts generated by the installation of the Amador Aguiar I and II plants (Capim Branco I and II) in the municipality of Uberlândia/MG. In: **Anais 5ª UFU Academic Week.** Available at: <http://www.ic- ufu.org/anaisufu2008/PDF/SA08-20301.PDF>. Accessed on: 04.03.2009.

ANNEX A

Table 1

List of birdlife recorded at the Amador Aguiar I and II HPPs, 2008.

TAXON NAME	POPULAR NAME	*STATUS* MIGRATORY
Struthioniformes Latham, 1790		
Rheidae Bonaparte, 1849		
Rhea americana (Linnaeus, 1758)	emu	R
Tinamiformes Huxley, 1872		
Tinamidae Gray, 1840		
Crypturellus undulatus (Temminck, 1815)	jackfruit	R
Crypturellus parvirostris (Wagler, 1827)	inhambu-chororó	R
Rhynchotus rufescens (Temminck, 1815)	partridge	R
Nothura maculosa (Temminck, 1815)	yellow quail	R
Anseriformes Linnaeus, 1758		
Anhimidae Stejneger, 1885		
Anhima cornuta (Linnaeus, 1766)	anhuma	R
Anatidae Leach, 1820		
Dendrocygna viduata (Linnaeus, 1766)	irerê	R
Cairina moschata (Linnaeus, 1758)	mallard	R
Sarkidiornis sylvicola Ihering & Ihering, 1907	mallard	R
Amazonetta brasiliensis (Gmelin, 1789)	red foot	R
Galliformes Linnaeus, 1758		
Cracidae Rafinesque, 1815		
Penelope superciliaris Temminck, 1815	jacupemba	R
Crax fasciolata Spix, 1825	curassow	R
Podicipediformes Fürbringer, 1888		
Podicipedidae Bonaparte, 1831		
Tachybaptus dominicus (Linnaeus, 1766)	merguhâo- small	R
Pelecaniformes Sharpe, 1891		
Phalacrocoracidae Reichenbach, 1849		
Phalacrocorax brasilianus (Gmelin, 1789)	biguà	R
Anhingidae Reichenbach, 1849		
Anhinga anhinga (Linnaeus, 1766)	biguatinga	R
Ciconiiformes Bonaparte, 1854		
Ardeidae Leach, 1820		
Tigrisoma lineatum (Boddaert, 1783)	socó-boi	R
Cochlearius cochlearius (Linnaeus, 1766)	arapapà	R
Nycticorax nycticorax (Linnaeus, 1758)	savacu	R
Butorides striata (Linnaeus, 1758)	punch	R
Bubulcus ibis (Linnaeus, 1758)	heron	R
Ardea cocoi Linnaeus, 1766	heron	R
TAXON NAME	POPULAR NAME	*STATUS* MIGRATORY
Ardea alba Linnaeus, 1758	great egret	R
Syrigma sibilatrix (Temminck, 1824)	mary janes	R
Pilherodius pileatus (Boddaert, 1783)	heron	R
Egretta thula (Molina, 1782)	little egret	R
Threskiornithidae Poche, 1904		
Mesembrinibis cayennensis (Gmelin, 1789)	coró-coró	R
Phimosus infuscatus (Lichtenstein, 1823)	naked-faced tapicuru	R
Theristicus caudatus (Boddaert, 1783)	curicaca	R

Platalea aja Linnaeus, 1758	spoonbill	R
Ciconiidae Sundevall, 1836		
Jabiru mycteria (Lichtenstein, 1819)	tuiuiù	R
Mycteria americana Linnaeus, 1758	dry-headed	R
Cathartiformes Seebohm, 1890		
Cathartidae Lafresnaye, 1839		
Cathartes aura (Linnaeus, 1758)	red-headed vulture	R
Cathartes burrovianus Cassin, 1845	yellow-headed vulture	R
Coragyps atratus (Bechstein, 1793)	black-headed vulture	R
Sarcoramphus papa (Linnaeus, 1758)	king vulture	R
Falconiformes Bonaparte, 1831		
Accipitridae Vigors, 1824		
Leptodon cayanensis (Latham, 1790)	gray-headed hawk	R
Chondrohierax uncinatus (Temminck, 1822)	snail	R
Gampsonyx swainsonii Vigors, 1825	little hawk	R
Elanus leucurus (Vieillot, 1818)	plume hawk	R
Rostrhamus sociabiHs (Vieillot, 1817)	snail hawk	R
Ictiniaplumbea (Gmelin, 1788)	sovi	R
Accipiter striatus Vieillot, 1808	hawk-miùdo	R
Accipiter bicolor (Vieillot, 1817)	gaviâo-bombachinha-grande	R
Geranospiza caerulescens (Vieillot, 1817)	hawk- stilt	R
Buteogallus urubitinga (Gmelin, 1788)	black hawk	R
Heterospizias meridionalis (Latham, 1790)	goat hawk	R
Harpyhaliaetus coronatus (Vieillot, 1817)	grey eagle	R
Busarellus nigricollis (Latham, 1790)	beautiful hawk	R
Rupornis magnirostris (Gmelin, 1788)	hawk-hawk	R
Buteo albicaudatus Vieillot, 1816	white-tailed hawk	R
Buteo nitidus (Latham, 1790)	stone hawk	R
Buteo brachyurus Vieillot, 1816	short-tailed hawk	R
TAXON NAME	POPULAR NAME	*STATUS* MIGRATORY
Spizaetus tyrannus (Wied, 1820)	hawk-monkey	R
Spizaetus ornatus (Daudin, 1800)	hawk	R
Falconidae Leach, 1820		
Caracara plancus (Miller, 1777)	caracarà	R
Milvago chimachima (Vieillot, 1816)	cuddler	R
Herpetotheres cachinnans (Linnaeus, 1758)	acauâ	R
Micrastur semitorquatus (Vieillot, 1817)	clock hawk	R
Falco sparverius Linnaeus, 1758	kiriquiri	R
Falco femoralis Temminck, 1822 Gruiformes Bonaparte, 1854	collared hawk	R
Rallidae Rafinesque, 1815		
Aramides cajanea (Statius Muller, 1776)	three-pot saracura	R
Laterallus viridis (Statius Muller, 1776)	sanà-castanha	R
Laterallus melanophaius (Vieillot, 1819)	sanà-parda	R
Porzana albicollis (Vieillot, 1819)	sanà-carijó	R
Pardirallus nigricans (Vieillot, 1819)	saracura-sanà	R
Gallinula chloropus (Linnaeus, 1758)	water chicken	R
Porphyrio martinica (Linnaeus, 1766)	water chicken - blue	R
Heliornithidae Gray, 1840		
Heliornis fulica (Boddaert, 1783)	caper	R
Cariamidae Bonaparte, 1850		
Cariama cristata (Linnaeus, 1766)	seriema	R

Charadriiformes Huxley, 1867		
Jacanidae Chenu & Des Murs, 1854		
Jacana jacana (Linnaeus, 1766)	jaçanà	R
Charadriidae Leach, 1820		
Vanellus chilensis (Molina, 1782)	kite	R
Scolopacidae Rafinesque, 1815		
Tringa solitaria Wilson, 1813	solitary torch	VN
Actitis macularius (Linnaeus, 1766)	spotted sandpiper	VN
Columbiformes Latham, 1790		
Columbidae Leach, 1820		
Columbina talpacoti (Temminck, 1811)	turtledove	R
Columbina squammata (Lesson, 1831)	fire-extinguished	R
Claravispretiosa (Ferrari-Perez, 1886)	blue pararu	R
Columba livia Gmelin, 1789	domestic pigeon	R
Patagioenas picazuro (Temminck, 1813)	pigeon	R
Patagioenas cayennensis (Bonnaterre, 1792)	wood pigeon	R
Zenaida auriculata (Des Murs, 1847)	band dove	R
Leptotila verreauxi Bonaparte, 1855	pigeon pea	R
Leptotila rufaxilla (Richard & Bernard, 1792)	jellyfish	R
Psittaciformes Wagler, 1830		
Psittacidae Rafinesque, 1815		
TAXON NAME	POPULAR NAME	*STATUS* MIGRATORY
Ara ararauna (Linnaeus, 1758)	hyacinth macaw	R
Orthopsittaca manilata (Boddaert, 1783)	yellow-faced maracana Buriti maracana (CBRO)	R
Diopsittaca nobilis (Linnaeus, 1758)	maracanâ- small	R
Aratinga leucophthalma (Statius Muller, 1776)	periquitâ- maracanâ	R
Aratinga auricapillus (Kuhl, 1820)	red-fronted jandaia	R, E
Aratinga aurea (Gmelin, 1788)	king parakeet	R
Forpus Xanthopterygius (Spix, 1824)	tuim	R
Brotogeris chiriri (Vieillot, 1818)	yellow-rumped parakeet	R
Alipiopsitta xanthops (Spix, 1824)	kite	R
Amazona aestiva (Linnaeus, 1758)	real parrot	R
Amazona amazonica (Linnaeus, 1766)	curica	R
Cuculiformes Wagler, 1830		
Cuculidae Leach, 1820		
Coccyzus melacoryphus Vieillot, 1817	fluted caterpillar	R
Piaya cayana (Linnaeus, 1766)	cat's soul	R
Crotophaga ani Linnaeus, 1758	black anu	R
Guira guira (Gmelin, 1788)	white anu	R
Tapera naevia (Linnaeus, 1766)	saci	R
Strigiformes Wagler, 1830		
Tytonidae Mathews, 1912		
Tyto alba (Scopoli, 1769)	church owl	R
Strigidae Leach, 1820		
Megascops choliba (Vieillot, 1817)	little owl	R
Pulsatrix perspicillata (Latham, 1790)	murucututu	R
Glaucidium brasilianum (Gmelin, 1788)	caburé	R
Athene cunicularia (Molina, 1782)	burrowing owl	R
Caprimulgiformes Ridgway, 1881		
Nyctibiidae Chenu & Des Murs, 1851		
Nyctibius griseus (Gmelin, 1789)	moon-mother	R

Caprimulgidae Vigors, 1825		
Lurocalis semiiorquaius (Gmelin, 1789)	tuju	R
Chordeiles pusillus Gould, 1861	bacurauzinho	R
Nyctidromus albicollis (Gmelin, 1789)	bacurau	R
Caprimulgus parvulus Gould, 1837	bacurau-chintâ	R
Hydropsalis torquata (Gmelin, 1789)	scissor booby	R
Apodiformes Peters, 1940		
Apodidae Olphe-Galliard, 1887		
Cypseloides senex (Temminck, 1826)	old taperuçu	R
Streptoprocne zonaris (Shaw, 1796)	white-collared taperuçu	R
TAXON NAME	POPULAR NAME	*STATUS* MIGRATORY
Chaetura meridionalis Hellmayr, 1907	storm swallow	R
Tachornis squamata (Cassin, 1853)	little scissors	R
Trochilidae Vigors, 1825		
Phaethornis pretrei (Lesson & Delattre, 1839)	fluted whitetail	R
Eupetomena macroura (Gmelin, 1788)	scissor hummingbird	R
Aphantochroa Cirrochloris (Vieillot, 1818)	gray hummingbird	R
Florisuga fusca (Vieillot, 1817)	black hummingbird	R
Colibri serrirostris (Vieillot, 1816)	violet-eared hummingbird	R
Anthracothorax nigricollis (Vieillot, 1817)	black-tailed hummingbird	R
Chlorostilbon aureoventris (d'Orbigny & Lafresnaye, 1838)	red beetle	R
Thalurania furcata (Gmelin, 1788)	green scissor hummingbird	R
Amazilia versicolor (Vieillot, 1818)	white-banded hummingbird	R
Amazilia fimbriata (Gmelin, 1788)	green-throated hummingbird	R
Heliomaster squamosus (Temminck, 1823)	white-banded black beak	R, E
Calliphlox amethystina (Boddaert, 1783)	star - amethyst	R
Trogoniformes A. O. U., 1886		
Trogonidae Lesson, 1828		
Trogon surrucura Vieillot, 1817	surucuâ-variado	R
Coraciiformes Forbes, 1844		
Alcedinidae Rafinesque, 1815		
Ceryle torquatus (Linnaeus, 1766)	kingfisher - large	R
Chloroceryle amazona (Latham, 1790)	green kingfisher	R
Chloroceryle americana (Gmelin, 1788)	kingfisher - small	R
Momotidae Gray, 1840		
Baryphthengus ruficapillus (Vieillot, 1818)	green jungle	R
Momotus momota (Linnaeus, 1766)	blue-crowned udu	R
Galbuliformes Fürbringer, 1888		
Galbulidae Vigors, 1825		
Galbula ruficauda Cuvier, 1816	red-tailed pineapple	R
Bucconidae Horsfield, 1821		
Nystalus chacuru (Vieilloy, 1816)	JOHN BOB	R
Nystalus maculatus (Gmelin, 1788)	old boy	R
Nonnula rubecula (Spix, 1824)	macuru	R
Monasa nigrifrons (Spix, 1824)	cry-wet	R
TAXON NAME	POPULAR NAME	*STATUS* MIGRATORY

	black	
Chelidoptera tenebrosa (Pallas, 1782)	little vulture	R
Piciformes Meyer & Wolf, 1810		
Ramphastidae Vigors, 1825		
Ramphastos toco Statius Muller, 1776	toucanuçu	R
Pteroglossus castanotis Gould, 1834	brown goshawk	R
Picidae Leach, 1820		
Picumnus albosquamatus d'Orbigny, 1840	dwarf scaled woodpecker	R
Melanerpes candidus (Otto, 1796)	white woodpecker	R
Veniliornis passerinus (Linnaeus, 1766)	little dwarf	R
Colaptes melanochloros (Gmelin, 1788)	barred green woodpecker	R
Colaptes campestris (Vieillot, 1818)	field woodpecker	R
Dryocopus lineatus (Linnaeus, 1766)	white-banded woodpecker	R
Campephilus melanoleucos (Gmelin, 1788)	red-cockaded woodpecker	R
Passeriformes Linné, 1758		
Melanopareiidae Irestedt, Fjeldsâ, Johansson & Ericson, 2002		
Melanopareia torquata (Wied, 1831)	collar slap	R
Thamnophilidae Swainson, 1824		
Taraba major (Vieillot, 1816)	choró-boi	R
Thamnophilus doliatus (Linnaeus, 1764)	brooding	R
Thamnophilus pelzelni Hellmayr, 1924	plateau shock	R,E
Thamnophilus caerulescens Vieillot, 1816	woodcock	R
Dysithamnus mentalis (Temminck, 1823)	smooth	R
Herpsilochmus atricapillus Pelzeln, 1868	black-hat whine	R
Herpsilochmus longirostris Pelzeln, 1868	peckish cry	R
Conopophagidae Sclater & Salvin, 1873		
Conopophaga lineata (Wied, 1831)	tooth sucker	R
Dendrocolaptidae Gray, 1840		
Sittasomus griseicapillus (Vieillot, 1818)	green arapaçu	R
Dendrocolaptes platyrostris Spix, 1825	great arapaçu	R
Lepidocolaptes angustirostris (Vieillot, 1818)	arapaçu-de- cerrado	R
Furnariidae Gray, 1840		
Furnarius rufus (Gmelin, 1788)	john-of-the-woods	R
Synallaxis frontalis Pelzeln, 1859	petrim	R
Synallaxis albescens Temminck, 1823	ui-pi	R
Synallaxis scutata Sclater, 1859	black star	R
Cranioleuca vulpina (Pelzeln, 1856)	remote from the river	R
TAXON NAME	POPULAR NAME	*STATUS* MIGRATORY
Certhiaxis Cinnamomeus (Gmelin, 1788)	curutié	R
Phacellodomus ruffrons (Wied, 1821)	JOHN	R
Phacellodomus ruber (Vieillot, 1817)	gravedigger	R
Anumbius annumbi (Vieillot, 1817)	whisper	R
Hylocryptus rectirostris (Wied, 1831)	barrier piercing	R
Lochmias nematura (Lichtenstein, 1823)	JOHN-NUT	R
Xenops rutilans Temminck, 1821	bico-virado- carijó	R
Tyrannidae Vigors, 1825		
Leptopogon amaurocephalus Tschudi, 1846	big-headed	R
Corythopis delalandi (Lesson, 1830)	snapper	R
Hemitriccus margaritaceiventer (d'Orbigny & Lafresnaye, 1837)	golden-eyed snipe	R
Poecilotriccus latirostris (Pelzeln, 1868)	brown-faced	R

	blacksmith	
Todirostrum cinereum (Linnaeus, 1766)	ferreirinho - clock	R
Phyllomyias fasciatus (Thunberg, 1822)	louse	R
Myiopagis gaimardii (d'Orbigny, 1839)	maria-pechim	R
Myiopagis caniceps (Swainson, 1835)	gray guaracava	R
Myiopagis viridicata (Vieillot, 1817)	orange-crested guaracava	R
Elaenia flavogaster (Thunberg, 1822)	yellow-bellied guaracava	R
Elaenia spectabilis Pelzeln, 1868	large guaracava	R
Elaenia parvirostris Pelzeln, 1868	short-billed guaracava	R
Elaenia cristata Pelzeln, 1868	uniform-topped guaracava	R
Elaenia chiriquensis Lawrence, 1865	chibum	R
Elaenia obscura (d'Orbigny & Lafresnaye, 1837)	toucan	R
Camptostoma obsoletum (Temminck, 1824)	giggle	R
Suiriri suiriri (Vieillot, 1818)	grey suiri	R
Phaeomyias murina (Spix, 1825)	luggage rack	R
Tolmomyias sulphurescens (Spix, 1825)	black-eared flatbill	R
Platyrinchus mystaceus Vieillot, 1818	duckling	R
Myiophobus fasciatus (Statius Muller, 1776)	filipe	R
Hirundinea ferruginea (Gmelin, 1788)	leather gibbon	R
Lathrotriccus euleri (Cabanis, 1868)	rusty	R
Cnemotriccus fuscatus (Wied, 1831)	guaracavuçu	R
Contopus cinereus (Spix, 1825)	gray flycatcher	R
Pyrocephalus rubinus (Boddaert, 1783)	prince	R
Knipolegus cyanirostris (Vieillot, 1818)	bluish-black mary janes	R
Knipolegus lophotes Boie, 1828	black plume mary	R
TAXON NAME	POPULAR NAME	*STATUS* MIGRATORY
Satrapa icterophrys (Vieillot, 1818)	little suiriri	R
Xolmis cinereus (Vieillot, 1816)	spring	R
Xolmis velatus (Lichtenstein, 1823)	white-bride	R
Gubernetes yetapa (Vieillot, 1818)	scissors	R
Fluvicola nengeta (Linnaeus, 1766)	masked laundress	R
Arundinicola Ieucocephala (Linnaeus, 1764)	little nun	R
Colonia colonus (Vieillot, 1818)	widow	R
Machetornis rixosa (Vieillot, 1819)	boar suiriri	R
Legatus leucophaius (Vieillot, 1818)	pirate flycatcher	R
Myiozetetes cayanensis (Linnaeus, 1766)	ferrugineous-winged warbler	R
Myiozetetes similis (Spix, 1825)	red bentevinho-de-penacho	R
Pitangus sulphuratus (Linnaeus, 1766)	bird	R
Philohydor lictor (Lichtenstein, 1823)	bentevizinho-do-brejo	R
Myiodynastes maculatus (Statius Muller, 1776)	wrens	R
Megarynchus pitangua (Linnaeus, 1766)	neinei	R
Empidonomus varius (Vieillot, 1818)	peitica	R
Griseotyrannus aurantioatrocristatus (d'Orbigny & Lafresnaye, 1837)	black-hat cockatoo	R
Tyrannus albogularis Burmeister, 1856	white-throated suiriri	R
Tyrannus melancholicus Vieillot, 1819	suiriri	R

Tyrannus savana Vieillot, 1808	little scissors	R
Casiornis rufus (Vieillot, 1816)	cannoneer	R
Myiarchus swainsoni Cabanis & Heine, 1859	irré	R
Myiarchus ferox (Gmelin, 1789)	mary janes	R
Myiarchus tyrannulus (Statius Muller, 1776)	rusty-tailed mary-horse	R
Cotingidae Bonaparte, 1849		
Phibalura flavirostris Vieillot, 1816	bush scissors	R
Pipridae Rafinesque, 1815		
Neopelmapallescens (Lafresnaye, 1853)	fruxu-do- cerradâo	R
Antilophia galeata (Lichtenstein, 1823)	little soldier	R
Pipra fasciicauda Hellmayr, 1906	orange uirapuru	R
Tityridae Gray, 1840		
Tityra inquisitor (Lichtenstein, 1823)	anambé - white - brown - cheeked	R
Tityra cayana (Linnaeus, 1766)	black-tailed anambé	R
Pachyramphus validus (Lichtenstein, 1823)	black-hatted cinnamon tree	R
TAXON NAME	POPULAR NAME	*STATUS* MIGRATORY
Pachyramphus polychopterus (Vieillot, 1818)	black shin	R
Vireonidae Swainson, 1837		
Cyclarhis gujanensis (Gmelin, 1789)	pitiguari	R
Vireo olivaceus (Linnaeus, 1766)	juruviara	R
Corvidae Leach, 1820		
Cyanocorax cristatellus (Temminck, 1823)	field hawk	R
Cyanocorax Cyanopogon (Wied, 1821)	kangaroo chough	R,E
Hirundinidae Rafinesque, 1815		
Tachycineta albiventer (Boddaert, 1783)	river swallow	R
Tachycineta leucorrhoa (Vieillot, 1817)	white-rumped swallow	R
Progne tapera (Vieillot, 1817)	field swallow	R
Progne chalybea (Gmelin, 1789)	domestic swallow	R
Pygochelidon cyanoleuca (Vieillot, 1817)	little house swallow	R
Atticora melanoleuca (Wied, 1820)	collared swallow	R
Alopochelidon fucata (Temminck, 1822)	swallow - brunette	R
Stelgidopteryx ruficollis (Vieillot, 1817)	sawyer swallow	R
Hirundo rustica Linnaeus, 1758	flock swallow	VN
Petrochelidon pyrrhonota (Vieillot, 1817)	ring-backed swallow	VN
Troglodytidae Swainson, 1831		
Troglodytes musculus Naumann, 1823	corruira	R
Thryothorus genibarbis Swainson, 1838	garrinchâo-father-grandfather	R
Thryothorus leucotis Lafresnaye, 1845	red-bellied garrinchâ	R
Donacobiidae Aleixo & Pacheco, 2006		
Donacobius atricapilla (Linnaeus, 1766)	japacanim	R
Polioptilidae Baird, 1858		
Polioptila dumicola (Vieillot, 1817	mask-tail scales	R
Turdidae Rafinesque, 1815		
Turdus subalaris (Seebohm, 1887)	sabià-ferreiro	R
Turdus rufiventris Vieillot, 1818	orange elderberry	R
Turdus leucomelas Vieillot, 1818	sabià-barranco	R
Turdus amaurochalinus Cabanis, 1850	sabià-poca	R
Mimidae Bonaparte, 1853		
Mimus saturninus (Lichtenstein, 1823)	field elder	R

Motacillidae Horsfield, 1821		
Anthus lutescens Pucheran, 1855	humming truck driver	R
Coerebidae d'Orbigny & Lafresnaye, 1838		
Coereba flaveola (Linnaeus, 1758)	cambacica	R
TAXON NAME	POPULAR NAME	*STATUS* MIGRATORY
Thraupidae Cabanis, 1847		
Schistochlamys melanopis (Latham, 1790)	collared sandpiper	R
Schistochlamys ruficapillus (Vieillot, 1817)	velvet beak	R,E
Cissopis leverianus (Gmelin, 1788)	tietinga	R
Neothraupis fasciata (Lichtenstein, 1823)	field cicada	R
Nemosia pileata (Boddaert, 1783)	black skunk	R
Thlypopsis sordida (d'Orbigny & Lafresnaye, 1837)	skirt-canary	R
Cypsnagra hirundinacea (Lesson, 1831)	flock	R
Eucometis penicillata (Spix, 1825)	kite	R
Tachyphonus coronatus (Vieillot, 1822)	black thieves	R
Tachyphonus rufus (Boddaert, 1783)	black kite	R
Ramphocelus carbo (Pallas, 1764)	red kite	R
Thraupis sayaca (Linnaeus, 1766)	grey sandpiper	R
Thraupis palmarum (Wied, 1823)	coconut sandpiper	R
Tangara cayana (Linnaeus, 1766)	yellow skirt	R
Tersina viridis (Illiger, 1811)	swallowtail	R
Dacnis cayana (Linnaeus, 1766)	blue skirt	R
Cyanerpes cyaneus (Linnaeus, 1766)	hummingbird skirt	R
Hemithraupis guira (Linnaeus, 1766)	black skirt	R
Conirostrum speciosum (Temminck, 1824)	brown arrowhead	R
Emberizidae Vigors, 1825		
Zonotrichia capensis (Statius Muller, 1776)	tico-tico	R
Ammodramus humeralis (Bosc, 1792)	field woodpecker	R
Sicalis citrina Pelzeln, 1870	dragon kite	R
Sicalis flaveola (Linnaeus, 1766)	true canary	R
Emberizoides herbicola (Vieillot, 1817)	field pigeon	R
Volatinia jacarina (Linnaeus, 1766)	tiziu	R
Sporophilaplumbea (Wied, 1830)	patativa	R
Sporophila collaris (Boddaert, 1783)	black collar	R
Sporophila lineola (Linnaeus, 1758)	mustache	R
Sporophila nigricollis (Vieillot, 1823)	Bahian	R
Sporophila caerulescens (Vieillot, 1823)	collar	R
Sporophila leucoptera (Vieillot, 1817)	crying	R
Sporophila angolensis (Linnaeus, 1766)	curio	R
Arremon flavirostris Swainson, 1838	yellow-billed woodpecker	R
Coryphospingus cucullatus (Statius Muller, 1776)	kinglet	R
Cardinalidae Ridgway, 1901		
Saltator maximus (Statius Muller, 1776)	viola seasoning	R
Saltator similis d'Orbigny & Lafresnaye,	iron-	R
TAXON NAME	POPULAR NAME	*STATUS* MIGRATORY
1837	true	
Saltator atricollis Vieillot, 1817	peppercorns	R
Cyanocompsa brissonii (Lichtenstein, 1823)	azure	R
Parulidae Wetmore, Friedmann, Lincoln, Miller, Peters, van Rossem, Van Tyne & Zimmer 1947		
Parula pitiayumi (Vieillot, 1817)	sissy	R

Geothlypis aequinoctialis (Gmelin, 1789)	snake	R
Basileuterus hypoleucus Bonaparte, 1830	white-bellied jumper	R
Basileuterus flaveolus (Baird, 1865)	wild canary	R
Basileuterus leucophrys Pelzeln, 1868	eyebrow jumper	R,E
Icteridae Vigors, 1825		
Psarocolius decumanus (Pallas, 1769)	japu	R
Cacicus haemorrhous (Linnaeus, 1766)	coon	R
Icterus cayanensis (Linnaeus, 1766)	meeting	R
Icterus jamacaii (Gmelin, 1788)	corruption	R,E
Gnorimopsar chopi (Vieillot, 1819)	graûna	R
Chrysomus ruficapillus (Vieillot, 1819)	garibaldi	R
Pseudoleistes guirahuro (Vieillot, 1819)	chopim-do-brejo	R
Molothrus oryzivorus (Gmelin, 1788)	iraûna-grande	R
Molothrus bonariensis (Gmelin, 1789)	turd	R
Sturnella superciliaris (Bonaparte, 1850)	police-inglesa-do-sul	R
Fringillidae Leach, 1820		
Carduelis magellanica (Vieillot, 1805)	goldfinch	R
Euphonia chlorotica (Linnaeus, 1766)	end-to-end	R
Passeridae Rafinesque, 1815		
Passer domesticus (Linnaeus, 1758)	sparrow	R

Source: MANNA AND TOLEDO (2008).

Migratory status: VN = seasonal visitor species from the northern hemisphere.

R = resident species. RE = endemic species.

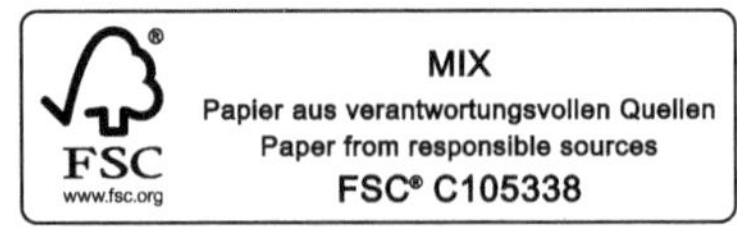

Printed by Books on Demand GmbH, Norderstedt / Germany